"*The Emotional Eating Workbook* is a delightful, informative, and passionate tour of the underpinnings of emotional eating. It is filled with timely and effective tools designed to end one's battle with food. As a reader-friendly text, it will serve as an important work in the treatment of emotional eating."

—**Ralph E. Carson, RD, PhD**, consultant for the Pine Grove Women's Center at Pine Grove Behavioral Health and Addiction Services in Hattiesburg, MS, and board member of The International Association of Eating Disorders Professionals

"*The Emotional Eating Workbook* nourishes body, mind, emotions, and spirit. Carolyn Ross's inspired and accessible program enhances mindful awareness, which leads to more natural, authentic, and skillful choices. If emotional eating is a problem for you, this book holds the keys to a breakthrough."

—**Joan Borysenko, PhD**, author of *The PlantPlus Diet Solution* and *Minding the Body, Mending the Mind*

"With compassion, wisdom, and creativity, Carolyn Ross's *The Emotional Eating Workbook* can open a pathway to healing for individuals struggling with the complex issue of emotional eating. Ross's approach looking at the core issues will help readers discover the underlying factors that drive their struggles with food. I highly recommend this valuable workbook!"

—**Wendy Oliver-Pyatt, MD, FAED, CEDS**, executive director of the Oliver-Pyatt Centers, www.oliverpyattcenters.com

THE
Emotional
Eating
WORKBOOK

A Proven-Effective,
Step-by-Step Guide to
End Your Battle with Food
& Satisfy Your Soul

CAROLYN COKER ROSS, MD, MPH

New Harbinger Publications, Inc.

Publisher's Note

This publication is designed to provide accurate and authoritative information in regard to the subject matter covered. It is sold with the understanding that the publisher is not engaged in rendering psychological, financial, legal, or other professional services. If expert assistance or counseling is needed, the services of a competent professional should be sought.

Distributed in Canada by Raincoast Books

Copyright © 2016 by Carolyn Coker Ross
          New Harbinger Publications, Inc.
          5674 Shattuck Avenue
          Oakland, CA 94609
          www.newharbinger.com

Cover design by Sara Christian

Acquired by Melissa Kirk

Edited by Gretel Hakanson

All Rights Reserved

Library of Congress Cataloging-in-Publication Data on file

Printed in the United States of America

21   20   19

10   9   8   7   6   5   4   3

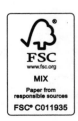

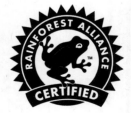

This book is dedicated to my sons Dutch and Sam and my granddaughter, Malia, for their inspiration and support. Finally my son Noah has continued to be a source of inspiration to me in all that I do both before and after his untimely death.

Contents

Acknowledgments

I would like to thank my agent, Chris Tomasino, who spent a lot of time and effort in the preparation of this book and continued to have faith in my writing and in the book project for two years before it even went to the publisher. Thanks also to my hardworking editors at New Harbinger, Jess Beebe and Melissa Kirk. I have had the pleasure now of completing two books with them, and I know that all their hard work has taken my writing to a better level.

Introduction

Food and weight issues and associated body image issues affect a large portion of the world's population. You may be one of the over 1.4 billion adults across the world (in 2008) who were overweight and more than half a billion who were considered obese (World Health Organization 2014). Even if you aren't overweight or obese, you may struggle with food issues such as food cravings, food fears, or compulsive overeating. You may also have body image issues in which you feel your body has betrayed you by not being the size or shape you'd want it to be, or for whatever reason, you may feel dissatisfied with your body. If any of that is true, you may be spending a lot of your time worrying about your appearance or body size, trying to lose weight or fighting not to regain weight you've lost, trying diets, worrying about shopping for clothes, and feeling ashamed of how you look. By now, you may have also realized that dieting doesn't work—at least not in the long run. If you are feeling hopeless or you feel as if nothing has really worked for you, then this book will make a lot of sense.

This book will help you understand why you've had such trouble with your weight. You will learn how your weight, food, and body image issues are connected to experiences you may have had as a child or adult, to your emotions, and to beliefs you've formed (usually unconsciously) about yourself and life that keep you stuck. But besides telling you the "why" of your food and weight issues, this book will provide you with ways to remove these blocks and also practical and sustainable solutions for the common pitfalls that most people with food, weight, and body image issues struggle with—issues such as how to stop emotional eating, deal with stress without food, and remove blocks to moving your body. Most importantly, you will learn to shift your focus about your food and body image issues and your weight from a place of dissatisfaction and nothing-ever-works hopelessness to one of reaching your goals by living to satisfy your soul, not the scale. This may seem like a foreign concept now, but just ask yourself why you *really* want to lose weight or why you are *really* dissatisfied with your body or why you *really* overeat or binge eat. Perhaps you, like many of the clients I work with who have these issues, secretly feel that if you could just be thin or just lose weight, then your life would work out. In fact, it's the other way around. If you can live with more joy in your life, reaching a healthy weight becomes less difficult. If this statement confuses you, this book will provide you with proof that what I'm saying really works.

In part 1, you will learn how to remove emotional blocks and shift any unhealthy beliefs you may have. You will learn more about the "whys" that got you to where you are today. This is essential because emotional blocks and unhealthy core beliefs contribute to your inability or difficulty maintaining progress in your goals to have a better body image, to have a healthy relationship with food, and to reach a healthy weight. In part 2, you will develop daily practices to reduce emotional eating, to be better at stress management, and to improve your ability to bring more mindful joy back into your life, which will have an effect on your eating as well as on other areas of your life. Finally, at the end of the book, you will be presented with a seven-week program that will help you incorporate all that you've learned into daily practices that will support you in reaching your goals.

This book is about hope. It is about helping you take your focus off the number on the scale and put it on what really underlies your ability, and what blocks that ability, to live the best, most authentic life you can live. This book is about the Anchor Program. It's about helping you find your own anchor. Finding your anchor is about living from your authentic self and accessing your inner strength. It's not about offering you another diet, because diets don't work. It's about offering you a life in which food is enjoyed but is not used for unhealthy reasons that impact your self-esteem, your weight, and your body image. If you are ready to really transform your relationship with food and your body, read on!

PART I

The Anchor Program's Five Levels of Healing

In the first five chapters of this book, you will learn about the five levels of healing:

- stopping surface behaviors

- emerging from the emotional soup

- embracing the wisdom of body sensations

- challenging core beliefs and embracing new guiding principles

- finding soul satisfaction

Going through each level will enable you to remove emotional blocks to reaching your heartfelt goal to heal your food and weight issues. If you've tried different diets to help with these issues, you may have come to the conclusion that your food and weight issues are not about food. These issues are about how you use food to deal with your emotions, experiences from your past, and beliefs that have resulted from past hurts or traumas. By working on your food and weight issues on a deeper level, you can expect your healing to also be deeper and more sustainable. As part of this, you will find yourself feeling more comfortable around food, more able to make your own decisions about what to eat and how much based on your body's wisdom, and able to replace limiting beliefs from your past with guiding principles that are more in line with who you truly are. Most importantly, you will find yourself more able to express your true, authentic self without having to worry about your size or what other people think of you. The Anchor Program described in this book is about being true to yourself and accessing your inner strength.

CHAPTER 1

Stopping Surface Behaviors: Why Diets Don't Work and Why It's Not About the Food

Billy had always been a "husky" kid. His parents were both somewhat overweight. Everyone thought that because of Billy's size, he would follow in his dad's footsteps and be a star football player in high school. When Billy was in fifth grade, his life took an unexpected turn—his mother died of breast cancer. After her death, he began to put on a lot of weight. By high school, he weighed over four hundred pounds. In desperation, he decided to have gastric bypass surgery to get the weight off. Initially he lost weight, but over time he found himself unable to stop bingeing despite his doctor telling him he could rupture his new post-surgical stomach. Within two years, he had regained the weight he'd lost. Treating the surface symptom—his weight—did not solve Billy's problem.

Healing food, weight, and body image issues, which are often lifelong, is not about just eating better food or being more active, no matter what the experts say. It requires an approach that takes you step-by-step through the parts of yourself that are responsible for the beginning and continuation of your struggles with weight, food, and body image issues: your behaviors, your emotions, your beliefs, and your relationship with your body and with food. The goal of taking these steps is for you to be able to "clean house," to remove the things that no longer fit your current life that may have been leftover from your past. In this chapter, we will address the behaviors that keep your weight and food issues in place and how to realign those behaviors with your authentic self and with how you want to live now.

Problems with food or weight are like an iceberg. Everyone can see the ice that is above the surface of the water, but they can't always see the larger part of the iceberg that's beneath the water. What gets everyone's attention is what's above the surface—weight, eating behaviors such as bingeing or overeating, and body dissatisfaction. These behaviors can make your life unmanageable, creating financial hardships, medical problems, and general unhappiness. Your food and body image problems and the associated behaviors are what gets everyone's attention because they are what you are focused on, what your friends and family know that you worry about, and what take over your life. Imagine what your life would be like if you didn't spend most of your time thinking about your weight, how to lose weight, what you look like, how ashamed you are of your body, what you're planning to eat or what you are trying to keep yourself from eating, and so on.

You may be reading this and thinking, *My weight is the most important problem. If I could just lose weight, I wouldn't have a problem.* If you put your focus on the number on the scale and all the behaviors you use to try to change that number, you will miss the opportunity for healing at the deepest level possible. True healing requires not only that you access what is on the surface but that you look for and heal the root cause of your food and weight issues, which usually lies beneath the surface (and is not as obvious). Weight and food issues are just signs of the bigger problem. For this reason, only addressing the weight or eating problem does not affect the deeper issues of emotions that may be out of control and cause you to overeat, of beliefs that are unconscious but are driving the eating behaviors, and of a lack of connection with your body's innate wisdom, which can help you with your eating and weight issues. A person can stop bingeing or purging but still be at the mercy of deeper beliefs, emotions, and preoccupations that take him away from all he truly wants in his life, including happiness and peace of mind. Beneath the surface are strong and sometimes painful emotions, core beliefs, and body sensations that drive these behaviors. These superficial behaviors are a way to keep these powerful and sometimes frightening emotions and beliefs at bay. For example, Billy used food as a way to cope with sadness and grief. Just as in Billy's case, only addressing the superficial layer with dieting or even bariatric surgery won't solve the underlying problems and will lead to the weight being regained.

Superficial Behaviors

The eating behaviors at the *superficial level* include overeating; bingeing; dieting; the use of diet pills, diuretics, or laxatives; purging; and emotional overeating. Other behaviors that can be put in this level are drug addiction, alcoholism, sex addiction, and love and relationship addiction. While these latter behaviors may not be specifically food related, they often co-occur with weight and body image issues.

The first step to healing is learning to stop the behaviors, which will give you the space to recover who you are (your authentic self) and to learn to understand and cope with troubling emotions in ways that don't involve food.

Changing Superficial Behaviors

Just as icebergs come in many shapes and sizes, you may find your reaction to addressing your weight, body image, and food problems will show up in many different forms. Sometimes what's on the surface seems so big and overwhelming ("How am I going to lose one hundred pounds?!") that you may feel like you are standing on the edge of a cliff and are terrified of jumping off. In other cases, what's on the surface may seem like something that isn't too hard to do ("I've lost weight before; I can do it again"), but when you start to look deeper—at what's beneath the surface, at the emotions driving your behaviors, at past hurts and traumas, or even at core beliefs you've held dear most of your life—you become fearful and overwhelmed and can't see a way through. Both reactions are normal and not unexpected.

You may also find that you have a dual or conflicted relationship with these behaviors. For example, you may recognize that certain foods don't make you feel good but that you can't stop eating them. You may binge on sugary foods in the afternoon, then feel sick and tired most of the rest of the day only to find yourself wanting to binge again later in the evening. Eating certain foods may be comforting but may result in feelings of guilt and shame afterwards. This is the dual relationship. As you work through this book, you will find other ways to comfort or nurture yourself. As part of preparing yourself to stop these behaviors, it will help you to become more aware of how food came to represent love, comfort, safety, or whatever it currently represents to you. Until you are able to identify the original connection that you forged with food, you will have difficulty breaking the cycle that keeps you stuck because your mind may think you want to eat because you are hungry while your emotions are driving you to eat because of long-lost memories connecting specific foods to love, comfort, or safety. This awareness will explain why you couldn't stop bingeing on certain foods or why you find yourself overeating to the point of feeling sick even though you don't really want to. As we go through the first five chapters, you will start making these connections.

Caution: If you find yourself feeling overwhelmed or stuck at any time during this process, you may need to reach for support. Support can come in the form of professional help from a therapist, or you may feel supported by reaching out to a friend or family member.

EXERCISE: **Identifying Your Behaviors**

Checkmark all the behaviors that may have some relationship to your weight or to how you feel about food and your body.

☐ bingeing (eating a large quantity of food in a short period of time, usually two hours or less)

☐ hiding or hoarding food

☐ eating in secret

☐ emotional eating

☐ overeating under stress

☐ overeating when tired

☐ using diet pills, laxatives, or water pills (diuretics)

☐ not eating all day (restricting)

☐ stealing food

☐ using illegal drugs to manage your appetite

☐ dieting

☐ other: _____

☐ other: _____

Do I Really Need to Eat That?

Everything you do, including your eating behaviors and why you eat what you eat, and how you feel about your body, happens for a reason. It's called the superficial level because while it is a problem, it is not the root cause—it's just what is closest to the surface. Food isn't the problem. It's how you use food that causes problems. If you only address behaviors, change will be temporary. It is necessary to dig deeper—to look beneath the surface—to understand what drives you to use food the way you do.

Often the behaviors that are part of the superficial level started when you were younger but only became disruptive as you got older. These behaviors may have been preceded by events in your life that you probably have not thought about in years and may not connect to your current problems with weight.

Life experiences play a key role in the development and perpetuation of eating and weight problems. Difficult life experiences can often cause confusion between eating for nourishment and eating just for pleasure. This can lead us to convince ourselves that we need to treat, reward, or comfort ourselves with food.

Eating behavior is controlled by the brain, which coordinates hunger and fullness cues with information sent from the digestive tract. One part of the brain (the hypothalamus) controls the *need* to eat for survival that is inherent in all living organisms. A different part of the brain controls our *desire* to eat. This part of the brain is called the dopamine reward center. Often the need to eat for survival can be overridden by our desire for a certain taste or a certain food. This is what can lead to obesity. In olden times, when food was harder to obtain and there were no fast-food restaurants, there was no obesity. If you lived during those times, you had just enough food to meet your body's needs but rarely more than that. In modern times, there is an abundance of food, and food is much more easily available. There are restaurants, fast-food places, grocery stores, and so on. So unless you live in a developing country or you are extremely poor, you will have enough food to eat. Eating beyond your need for food usually means eating comfort foods that are often high in sugar, fat, and salt. These foods are eaten not for their nutritional value but for their taste, to satisfy emotional cravings, or to cope with stress. There is nothing wrong with eating tasty treats, but your inability to forego these foods or to stop compulsively overeating them is a sign you may be using such foods not just for their taste but for emotional reasons. People consume these foods even when they are not hungry and often without thinking about what they are eating and sometimes without even enjoying what they are eating. It is important to interrupt this cycle in order to manage your weight.

EXERCISE: Identifying Trigger Foods and Their Emotional Connections

Make a list below of foods you tend to eat out of want, out of desire or craving, or as a reward. These will usually be the same foods you binge on or overeat.

1. _____

2. _____

3. _____

4. _____

5. _____

Now, describe why you eat each of these specific foods. What is the feeling, taste, and texture of the food you binge on or overeat the most? Write at least a paragraph about what each of your comfort foods means to you.

_____

_____

_____

_____

_____

List below any insights that explain why "it's not about the food." What would be missing in your life if you no longer could turn to these specific foods to deal with your problems or your emotions? Notice any descriptions in the paragraph above that are clues to the purpose food serves for you and list them below. *(Example: If I couldn't turn to food, I would miss the immediate comfort I get from eating my favorite foods.)*

_____

_____

_____

_____

Why Diets Don't Work

If you are overweight, you may be motivated to diet and lose weight for many important reasons—for better health and well-being, for increased mobility, to be more socially accepted, and to avoid being teased or bullied about your weight. You may also believe that losing weight will solve other problems in your life, such as feeling isolated, wanting a relationship, or wanting to get ahead at work. Losing weight can produce a temporary feeling of happiness only to be replaced by self-blame, despair, or depression when you are not able to maintain your weight loss. It has become part of our culture to use diets to lose weight and when they don't work, to blame ourselves for "not sticking with it."

Despite the fact that studies show diets don't result in sustainable weight loss, you may be like the majority of overweight individuals who still believe that dieting is an effective weight loss strategy (Thomas et al. 2008). Not only do diets not work, but if you've been dieting off and on throughout your life, you may have noticed, as one study shows, that you've regained more weight than you've lost, which is the experience of two-thirds of dieters in studies (Mann et al. 2007). One of the problems that many heavy individuals face is that they've been told over and over that if they don't lose weight, they cannot be healthy. While this may be a temporary motivator that has helped you diet in the past, having the focus on your weight doesn't necessarily change your health. You are more likely to improve your health if you focus on changing your behaviors, rather than on the number on the scale. Studies support that when you put your focus on health first, not weight, you're more likely to improve your health, self-esteem, and body image and lower your risk for heart disease, high blood pressure, and diabetes through size acceptance, intuitive eating, and increased activity levels (Bacon and Aphramor 2011).

If it's clear that diets don't work, why do most people keep turning to the latest fad diet, hoping that each time things will be different? The answer is that each diet represents a hope they have of changing their life. In our fat-phobic, diet-obsessed culture, we have come to confuse being thin with being happy. We have been conditioned to believe that we have to look a certain way in order to deserve the life we want. We have been taught by the media, our families, and society that if we are in a bigger body—or if we are different in any way from what society deems acceptable (young, thin, not gay, of a certain race or religion or political affiliation)—that we cannot have what others have and, most importantly, what we desperately want.

Each of us has within us a longing for our best life, for our dream life. What is confusing is that we have equated superficial qualities of appearance and size, for example, with what they represent for us in our best life. For example, if you believe you have to be thin in order to have the relationship you long for, you may have forgotten what you're really longing for, which is the feeling of intimate connection and how that would fill your heart. If you have not been able to reach your weight goal, you may have closed yourself to any chance of that happening unless and until you are thin. In essence, dreams are postponed or even shut down, waiting for you to have your perfect body. In the next exercise, you'll list the dreams you've been putting on hold until you are thin.

EXERCISE: **What Have Your Food and Weight Issues Cost You?**

Make a list of your postponed dreams and how postponing them has affected you emotionally, physically, and spiritually.

The dreams I've put on hold:	What putting this dream on hold has cost me emotionally, physically, and spiritually:

Whenever you put your dreams on hold, waiting for a certain thing to happen, you are saying (sometimes unconsciously) that they won't matter unless they show up in a certain package. You are essentially saying that *you* don't matter enough to have the life you deserve.

Most of us have some box that we live in that is limiting. It is our own personal prison. Usually our boxes are filled with judgments from the past and fears about the future. It may be the box of "If only I had more money, then I would _____." Or your box may have to do with not having enough education or family support. But in the bigger scheme of things, life is meant to be about moving through our limits and learning to live the life we were born to live. This is the life our authentic self is calling us to live. It is the life where fear does not hold eminent domain, where embarrassment or shame can't stop us from doing the things we love, and where ultimately we step into our authentic self's passion for just *being the best we can be*. Does that sound far-fetched? Not achievable? Impossible? Well it isn't. It is about taking a journey of *self*-discovery where your weight is not an unreasonable burden to be shed like an old coat. On this journey your weight becomes your portal to self-awakening.

When you've tried all the diets that have promised the impossible, when you've come to realize that you are not happy living in the box that society and your own past conditioning have put you into, and when you are ready to live with courage and have a desire to heal, then you are ready to move deeper, where you will discover your anchor—your own true self. It's not about taking a big leap but rather about taking a series of next steps.

In the next chapter, your first step awaits you: the opportunity to explore how emotions can influence your behaviors and your weight.

CHAPTER 2

Emerging from the Emotional Soup

Maryann just turned sixty years old. She is married and has a successful career in nursing. Although she feels good about most things in her life, she continues to struggle with her weight. When she feels happy, she overeats. When she's sad or angry, she overeats. When her husband has to work late and she's home alone, she overeats. She describes food as "my best friend." Even though she has read many diet books and has been on numerous fad diets, she can't seem to stop herself from having a "few more cookies." A few more always leads to half a bag or a whole bag. Then the guilt comes, and she feels ashamed at having so little control. She feels that she is a weak person and is embarrassed that she is not able to control herself. She compares herself to her mother, who is very overweight, and she can't stand to think that she's turned out to be like her. Throughout her childhood, Maryann remembers her mother constantly telling her what to eat and what not to eat and that if she didn't lose weight, she'd never get married. Her husband is very health conscious and often makes disparaging comments about her weight. She feels disappointed in her inability to control her weight. She really believes that if her life were just less stressful, she could stop overeating. Or if her husband were more affectionate, she wouldn't turn to food for comfort.

In this chapter, you will learn about the hidden force that is driving your behaviors and what you can do to uncouple your behaviors from the emotions that drive them. These emotional drivers come from past experiences and beliefs, from old traumas that have never healed, and from current experiences that replicate old emotional patterns. You will also learn to identify emotional responses that are not congruent with whom you are today. Part of changing your behaviors is understanding the deeper driving forces behind them. Once you become aware of how emotions can trigger the behaviors you identified in chapter 1, you will have a better chance of responding to your emotions in a way that doesn't involve using food to numb yourself from the pain of your emotions, shove them down, or ignore them. In this chapter, you will also learn about emotional patterns that may have originated in childhood and how those may be affecting your current-day reactions. Maryann's story above, for example, demonstrates how people in her life, starting with her mother and now her husband, have focused on her weight. The emotions she feels about this started in her childhood, and now, as an adult, these same emotions are triggered when her husband makes comments about her weight or lack of fitness. The emotions of embarrassment, guilt, shame, anger, loneliness, and disappointment are the driving force behind her overeating.

If you are like many people with food and weight issues, you may be able to recognize that your emotions at times feel overwhelming, or you may be the type of person who has completely shut down any access to your emotions and even has trouble identifying what you are feeling. Both reactions to emotional pain are two sides of the same coin—attempts to escape from your emotions, or from the "emotional soup." When you are stuck in the emotional soup, you may feel that your emotions are in charge of you as opposed to the other way around. Emerging from the emotional soup requires emotional development— that is, being able to identify, express, understand, and very importantly, regulate your emotions. It is not your emotions themselves that cause problems in your life. Rather it is your attempt to suppress or avoid your emotions that leads to problems. When emotions are not acknowledged, they find expression in the foods you eat, in the size and shape of your body, and in the need to eat foods that may be soothing momentarily but don't quench the soul's hunger for expression. Emotional regulation means being able to cope with emotions without resorting to unhealthy or self-defeating behaviors. Many factors that influence emotional development and especially emotional regulation will be discussed in this chapter. But first, I'd like to talk about what emotions are and why they are so important in our lives.

What Are Emotions?

Emotions can be defined as "internal phenomena that can, but do not always, make themselves observable through expression and behavior" (Niedenthal, Krauth-Gruber, and Ric 2006, 5). Webster's dictionary defines an emotion as "a conscious mental reaction (as anger or fear) subjectively experienced as strong feeling usually directed toward a specific object and typically accompanied by physiological and behavioral changes in the body" (Merriam-Webster Online, s.v. "emotion"). The Taoist view of emotions is that they are energy. Emotions can be called the energy of self-expression. How we express ourselves emotionally becomes part of how others identify us and often how we think of ourselves. Emotions can also influence our perceptions. For example, if you hear a dog barking, depending on your past experience and perception of dogs, you may try to pet the dog. If on the other hand, your past experiences with dogs have been negative and led to a fear of dogs or if the dog seems threatening, you may want to avoid getting close to the dog. Emotions can be the signal that can draw us toward what we like and warn us away from danger. In the case of a dog barking, perception partly determines how you view the situation. But the emotion of fear at the sound of a dog barking can also be a sign of true danger. The tricky part is sorting out what is perception and what is real danger. Often past experiences make it difficult for us to see what is real, and in this chapter you will learn more about the impact of experience on perception and how it can color reality.

Emotions can also help you make decisions in your life. People who have had damage to the emotional parts of the brain find it difficult, if not impossible, to make decisions. If you have had damage to your emotional brain, you may have trouble making even simple decisions, such as what to eat (Bechara, Damasio, and Damasio 2000).

Humans and most other animals are equipped with a basic set of core emotions: fear, anger, surprise, disgust, joy, and sadness (Ekman, Friesen, and Ellsworth 1982). Humans also have a set of higher moral emotions that are dependent on our level of self-consciousness and ability to empathize with others. These include guilt, embarrassment, shame, and pride (Leary and Price 2012).

Later in this chapter, I will discuss emotional regulation at length. But next, I'd like to concentrate on the other aspects of emotional development—the ability to identify, accept, and express your emotions.

Identifying Emotions

There are many ways in which we are able to recognize emotions in ourselves and in others. Babies communicate their emotions nonverbally from birth through crying, facial expressions, and body postures. When a parent reads these nonverbal cues and responds appropriately, it creates a feeling of security and safety for the infant. Learning how to identify emotions in others happens when we are very young. How each of us learns to identify emotions varies greatly. As a child, you may have been taught about emotions through conversations about upsetting situations. For example, if you came home from school and your mother saw you were upset, she may have asked you to identify your emotions: "Jimmy, are you angry about something that happened at school?" However, you may have grown up in a home where when you came home from school upset, nobody paid attention or you were told, "Stop pouting and go to your room." If so, you may have learned that your emotions don't matter. If you were mistreated or abused as a child, you may have learned to be afraid of your emotions because showing emotions could lead to further abuse. Additionally, emotions may have been frightening to you as a child if you have a genetic predisposition to having very intense emotional responses or to being very sensitive to your own or others' emotions.

If you are not able to identify your emotions or the emotions of others, you may find yourself in situations that are dangerous. For example, if a bell goes off in school, the teacher shows that she is afraid, and the other kids begin to feel fear too, but you don't pick up on the cue, you may not realize that you need to exit the building quickly because of a fire. Another reason why it's important to identify your emotions is that otherwise you won't have a way to name your internal experience. You may feel awful but not know why and not be able to clearly express what "awful" means to you. Does feeling awful mean you're afraid or tired? Or does it mean you're depressed? Being able to identify your emotions is part of what allows you to express yourself as an individual. Finally, if you have been genetically predisposed to having very intense emotions but can't identify what you are feeling, you may feel overwhelmed by them and just shut down or numb yourself—with food, for example.

Facial expressions are a very important nonverbal way to identify emotions. The expressions used to convey seven universal emotions—anger, sadness, surprise, contempt, disgust, fear, and joy—are similar throughout the world (Matsumoto et al. 2008). In Western culture, scientists have been able to map twenty-one emotions that people use almost the exact same facial expressions for, including combination emotions such as "happily surprised" (Du, Tao, and Martinez 2014). Other nonverbal emotional cues can include body posture and hand gestures. If you are obese, you may also have had trouble recognizing nonverbal cues of emotions from others or lack the ability to describe and identify your own emotions, a condition called alexithymia, which tends to be higher in obese children and adults and women with binge-eating disorder (Baldaro et al. 2003; Pinaquy et al. 2003). What this means is that obese women who have difficulty communicating their feelings also are more likely to eat in response to their emotions. The exact causes of alexithymia are not known, but it may be the result of childhood abuse or may come about as a defense mechanism, a way of coping with previous experiences of intense and overwhelming emotional experiences (McDougall 1989).

Inability to identify emotions in oneself or others may also be a cause of emotional overeating, especially in men (Larsen et al. 2006). If you are a woman, you are probably more accurate than most men at identifying emotions from nonverbal cues such as facial expressions. It may be that women are socialized at an earlier age to identify nonverbal emotional cues, or it may be that the female brain is just programmed for this skill (Hall and Matsumoto 2004). There is a range of ways to express yourself emotionally. Some are healthier than others. But before you can express your emotions, you must become more aware of them. You must be able to identify what emotion you are feeling. In the exercise below, spend some time learning to identify your emotions.

EXERCISE: **Identifying Your Emotions**

In this exercise, you will identify specific emotions and their body sensations. Next to some of the emotions, I have listed common body locations for sensations associated with the emotion (Hendricks and Hendricks 1993) to help you get started. Start by listing a situation when you remember feeling each emotion strongly. Then list the body location and sensations associated with each emotion. Finally, see if you can identify nonverbal cues that are associated with each emotion. For example, think of your facial expressions, body posture, hand gestures, and other body language that indicate what you're feeling.

1. **Sadness**

   Situation: _____

   _____

Body location and sensations: *(Example: lump in throat, pressure in chest)*

_____

_____

Nonverbal signs: _____

_____

2. **Joy**

Situation: _____

_____

Body location and sensations: *(Example: chest area expansiveness, tingling in body)*

_____

_____

Nonverbal signs:_____

_____

3. **Anger**

Situation: _____

_____

Body location and sensations: *(Example: neck tension, clenched jaw, throbbing headache)*

_____

_____

Nonverbal signs:_____

_____

4. **Fear**

Situation: _____

_____

Body location and sensations: _____

_____

Nonverbal signs: _____

_____

5. **Shame**

Situation: _____

_____

Body location and sensations: _____

_____

Nonverbal signs: _____

_____

6. **Guilt**

Situation: _____

_____

Body location and sensations: _____

_____

Nonverbal signs: _____

_____

If you had trouble with this exercise, you will learn more about this important skill in upcoming chapters. For now, keep using the format above to track your emotions. Pay special attention to your body sensations as a clue to help you identify your emotions. Ask yourself: *What am I feeling? What is this emotion telling me about the situation I'm in?* Write down three emotions you experience each day using the format in this exercise. Do this for one month. You can record your insights in a journal on a daily basis or at the very least identify any strong emotions that come up over the next few weeks.

Emotional Expression

Learning to identify your emotions, to put a name to what you are feeling, is the first step to being able to express emotions in a healthy and safe way. Emotional expression is important because it allows you to be the individual you are, with your own perceptions, emotions, and viewpoints. Emotional expression also is a necessary part of what it means to be human.

Even if you didn't grow up in a dysfunctional home, the messages you learned about how to handle your emotions—for example which emotions were considered appropriate in which situations—may have come from your family's cultural background. There may have also been cultural rules about the kinds of events in which emotional expression was sanctioned. In many cultures, for example, crying as an expression of grief over the death of a loved one is considered normal.

Patterns of emotional expression may also be similar to patterns in your relationship with food. For example, you may skip meals (similar to withholding emotions), which usually sets you up for the next binge (or emotional outburst).

Many people have trouble expressing certain emotions—usually because they have a judgment about themselves (or feel others will judge them) if they feel certain feelings. For example, you may feel that you will be judged as being weak if you express sadness. Emotional expression must go hand in hand with emotional regulation, which you will learn about later in this chapter. For now, in the exercise below, see if you can find any links to your eating behaviors and your emotions.

EXERCISE: **How Do I Express My Emotions?**

1. Checkmark the emotions you have the most difficulty expressing, and write down the judgments you have about expressing these emotions or your fear of how others will judge you if you show certain feelings. (Note: The judgments you have when you express one of these emotions may lead to another emotion. For example, if you find yourself expressing anger, you may then feel ashamed that you lashed out in anger at a loved one. You should consider the anger and the subsequent shame and describe how you feel about both.)

☐ Anger

My judgment about expressing this emotion is: _____

_____

☐ Sadness/grief

My judgment about expressing this emotion is: _____

_____

☐ Fear

My judgment about expressing this emotion is: _____

_____

☐ Joy

My judgment about expressing this emotion is: _____

_____

☐ Guilt

My judgment about expressing this emotion is: _____

_____

☐ Shame

My judgment about expressing this emotion is: _____

_____

☐ Anxiety/nervousness

My judgment about expressing this emotion is: _____

_____

☐ Other: _____

My judgment about expressing this emotion is: _____

_____

2. For the emotions you have trouble expressing, list what you do when you feel that emotion. (*Example: When I feel sad, I tend to go somewhere alone and eat. I isolate myself.*)

When I feel _____,

I tend to _____

_____

When I feel _____,

I tend to _____

_____

When I feel _____,

I tend to _____

_____

When I feel _____,

I tend to _____

_____

3. Now ask yourself what would change for you if the judgments you expressed above were not "real." (For example: What if people who are sad are *not* weak? How would that change how you express your emotions?)

Emotion: _____

What would change? _____

_____

Emotion: _____

What would change? _____

_____

Emotion: _____

What would change? _____

_____

Emotion: _____

What would change? _____

_____

Emotion: _____

What would change? _____

_____

4. Try to reveal similarities between your food and weight issues and your emotional expression by answering the following questions.

   a. Does expressing your emotions more fully affect your eating behaviors?

   _____

   _____

   _____

   _____

   _____

   _____

   b. What happens to your relationship with food when you hold back your emotions or when you have an emotional explosion?

   _____

   _____

   _____

   _____

   _____

   c. Think of times when you've expressed your emotions in healthy ways and unhealthy ways, and ask yourself how each affects your eating.

   _____

   _____

   _____

   _____

   _____

   _____

How Did You Learn to Express Your Emotions?

Each family has patterns, often unspoken, concerning emotions. You may not remember specific rules being talked about, but the rules were the way you learned how to express your emotions—either directly or indirectly. Emotional rules can include ones that (1) allow a child to change his or her expression of certain emotions to protect another person's feelings and (2) mask emotions to protect himself or herself from harm or to avoid embarrassment (Saarni 1999). For example, your mother may not have told you not to get angry, but she may have left the room or given you a disapproving look whenever you expressed anger, indicating that expressing anger was unacceptable. Or your father may have yelled at you, "Don't you talk back to me," when you got angry, suggesting that it was not okay for you to get angry or express that anger, but that it was okay for him to do so.

EXERCISE: Your Family's Emotional Rules

1. Choose from the list below the family rules you learned growing up about emotional expression.

    ☐ Other people's feelings are more important than your own.

    ☐ Don't show any emotions that hurt someone else.

    ☐ Hide your anger.

    ☐ Keep your emotions to yourself.

    ☐ Use anger when you want to get attention.

    ☐ Ignore your feelings.

    ☐ Don't trust your emotions; trusting your logical mind is more reliable.

    ☐ Be happy even when you're not.

    ☐ Other: _____

    _____

2. How did what you learned from your family shape how you express emotions? (*Example: My dad was a rager. For me, expressing strong emotions is very scary. I don't like it when other people express strong emotions either. So I never let anyone see me angry.*)

_____

_____

_____

It's important to notice that emotions themselves are not bad or wrong. Sometimes messages you learn growing up may lead you to either follow family rules about emotions or turn against them reflexively. You may also have judgments about past experiences and the emotions associated with those experiences. These judgments and associated emotions are what keep you stuck in a story (experience) from your past. Re-experiencing the emotions that are kept in place by your judgment of past experiences is a cause of overeating and bingeing. For example, if you were angry at your ex-husband during your divorce proceedings, you may have a judgment that he is an awful person or a "jerk" because he hurt you. Every time you see him, that judgment may come up for you—"he's a jerk"—and you may feel angry and hurt all over again. If you hold on to this judgment and continue to stay angry about what happened during that time, you are stuck in a past that no longer exists in the present moment. You may feel very justified about your anger because your ex-husband did something that hurt you. But ask yourself whom your judgment and your anger toward him are really hurting. Are they hurting him? Probably not. They are hurting you. They are causing suffering for you. When you continue to go back and live in a past experience as if it's occurring in your present, it will have an effect on many areas of your life and your relationships—not just with your ex-husband but probably with other people in your life who may remind you of him or remind you of how he made you feel. Holding on to judgments about past experiences can also affect your desire to overeat as a way to numb a feeling that is really a relic from your past. If you think about it, you are not the same person who went through that experience, and holding on to it only contributes to suffering (and probably overeating or bingeing) now. To release yourself from the anger and hurts of the past, you have to stop judging your ex-husband. That is not to say you ignore your hurt feelings; rather, you remind yourself that the hurt is from the past, and you find ways, perhaps in therapy, to work through past hurts so you can live more fully in the present. When you hold on to the judgment, "He's a bad person because he hurt me," for example, you keep yourself imprisoned by the emotions associated with that old situation, rather than being the observer and actor in your present life. Doing this is not easy, but when you are able to see that holding on to the past only hurts you, you may find that it becomes more important for you to move through the past and live in the present. By releasing yourself from these judgments, you may find yourself more open to the full range of emotional expression available to us as human beings.

Emotional Regulation

In order to make the best use of emotions, it is important to know how to manage or regulate them without using food. Maryann's story above is a good example of an emotional overeater—someone who uses food to regulate her emotions.

Emotional regulation begins in early infancy when babies learn to self-soothe or calm themselves. Some 20 percent of babies show signs of difficulty with self-regulation through excessive crying, sleep, and feeding problems or attentional disorders (Schmid et al. 2010). For most, this is a temporary problem. But for some, this may be a sign of things to come. By the age of four, children have usually learned to change how they express emotions to suit the expectations of others—they've learned the cultural and family rules about emotional expression as discussed above. Most children continue to learn various self-regulation skills as they get older. They may learn, for example, to express negative emotions more often to their mother than their father, who may react more negatively to emotional displays. They may learn to distract themselves by running on the playground when they feel anxious.

You may be using many healthy ways of regulating your emotions in other areas of your life but, like Maryann, find yourself at a loss about to how to do that with weight, body dissatisfaction, and food issues. For example, Maryann has to regulate her emotions in her work as a nurse, where it may not be appropriate for her to express how she feels to her patients, but she can express those feelings to a coworker. While everyone overeats from time to time (Thanksgiving, for example), when you use food as your primary way of dealing with your emotions, it can not only exacerbate negative emotions, such as guilt and shame, but also lead to weight gain and subsequent body dissatisfaction. Part of what you will learn in this book is how to regulate your emotions so you don't have to use food as an unhealthy way of dealing with them. The goal is to be able to experience a normal range of emotions without feeling so uncomfortable with those emotions that you use food (or other substances or behaviors) to avoid dealing with them.

Why Is Emotional Regulation Important?

Emotional overeating behaviors are the result of poor emotional regulation strategies and skills, including the ability to identify and cope with emotions (Haedt-Matt and Keel 2011; Ricca et al. 2009). If you are an emotional overeater, this problem probably began early in your life. As a child, if you had trouble managing your emotions, this was a sign that you were at higher risk for being overweight or obese as an adult. Or if you had difficulty postponing gratification as a child, threw tantrums, or expressed excessive anger about food, this also would have put you at risk for weight and food issues (Agras et al. 2004; Seeyave et al. 2009).

Interestingly, if you are a person who has difficulty just accepting your feelings and being emotionally upset makes it hard for you to concentrate, focus, complete tasks, or work duties, you may also be more likely to struggle with food and weight issues (Gianini, White, and Masheb 2013; Sim and Zeman 2006). When your emotions are in charge, the consequences can be grave—for your relationships and certainly for your relationship with food and your body.

While eating in response to emotional triggers or negative moods is common in many with weight problems, you may have noticed that the negative emotions don't go away after you binge or overeat. Overeating may unconsciously be your way of trying to change those negative feelings. But ask yourself how long you get relief after a binge or after emotionally overeating. You may start out eating in response to anger only to find your anger still there after your binge. Only now, you're angry with yourself for eating that bag of chips! On top of that, you may then feel embarrassed and guilty about the binge. The point is using food to manage emotions is just not the most effective strategy. It may have been something you learned when you were a child and didn't really have other skills, but now you do, and you will learn to tap into other skill sets for emotional regulation.

To determine if you are an emotional overeater, complete the exercise below.

EXERCISE: **Are You an Emotional Overeater?**

Check the statements that apply to you.

☐ I tend to overeat when I am celebrating.

☐ I experience food cravings on a regular basis.

☐ I tend to eat certain foods whenever I am anxious, depressed, or my feelings are hurt.

☐ I use food to help me cope with emotional situations.

☐ Food is comforting to me.

☐ I tend to overeat when I am angry or upset.

☐ When I am worried about something, I want to overeat.

☐ Frequently, I overeat when I'm bored or lonely.

☐ When I'm in a good mood, I don't worry about what I eat.

☐ I often overeat when I'm angry at someone "just to show them they can't control me."

☐ I tend to overeat when I'm alone; I eat much less than I want when I'm with other people.

If you checked off three or more of the above signs, you are probably an emotional overeater. You will learn more about why you emotionally overeat or binge in the rest of this chapter.

Why Can't I Manage My Emotions?

Many individuals with weight problems or eating disorders learn at a very young age to suppress all or certain emotions. You may have been taught this directly, or you may have learned this message indirectly through experience or observation. If every time you got upset as a child you were told, "Be a good girl," or "Boys don't cry," over time you may have taken for granted that this is how you should behave. Or you may have had a parent who was a raging alcoholic and frightened you. This could lead you to avoid expressing your anger because you may be afraid of becoming like your alcoholic parent. This childhood experience can show up in adulthood as a fear of anyone who expresses anger, even if it's a healthy expression of anger by your spouse. This in turn could lead to avoiding any conflict in your relationship, which is not healthy for you. Another scenario in this situation is the child who identifies with and emulates the alcoholic parent, seeing him or her as the stronger parent. This could lead to an acceptance of raging as the way to show strength in relationships. In adulthood, she may become the person who rages, just as her father or mother did when she was growing up.

Another reason you may have difficulty with your emotions may have to do with specific types of experiences from your childhood, according to the Adverse Childhood Experiences (ACE) Study. If you experienced verbal, physical, or sexual abuse, if a member of your family was in jail, if one of your parents was mentally ill or abusing drugs or alcohol, or if your parents were divorced or your mother was a victim of domestic violence, your risk of having a weight problem (defined as having a body mass index [BMI] greater than or equal to 35kg/m^2) may be 46 percent higher than it is for people who did not have these detrimental childhood experiences (Brown et al. 2009; Felitti et al. 1998). One of the researchers in this study learned that "many of his patients had been unconsciously using obesity as a shield against unwanted sexual attention or as a form of defense against physical attack, and that many of them had been sexually and/or physically abused as children. That is to say, although obesity was conventionally viewed as the problem, it was often found to be the unconscious solution to other, far more concealed, problems" (see http://www.acestudy.org for more information; Anda and Felitti 2003, 1).

Abuse or neglect or any of the above negative experiences in childhood leads to what is called toxic stress. Toxic stress leads to an overproduction of the stress hormones, cortisol, adrenaline, and noradrenaline. This leads to physical damage to the brain. If you were a child who experienced toxic stress, then you lived your life in fight-flight-or-freeze mode. Everything in the world may have seemed dangerous or unsafe to you. This could have caused you to struggle or fall behind in school and have trouble developing healthy relationships with peers and teachers due to your inability to trust others, or you may have experienced a sense of underlying despair and frustration throughout your life. People who have had toxic stress in their life often find solace in food, drugs, or alcohol; inappropriate sex; high-risk sports; or work as a way to cope with their feelings of depression, fear, and shame. That is why overeating and obesity are not about food or about weight. Rather, the weight and overeating are a solution that you used when you were younger and didn't have the skills you have now, but they are not the problem. The problem has to do with toxic stress and what caused it.

Attachment Style and Expressing Emotions

Research is now showing that something called "attachment styles" may also explain why people with a history of toxic stress related to childhood trauma or to other specific childhood issues (abandonment, neglect, abrupt separation from a parent, frequent changes in caregivers, or lack of caregiver responsiveness) may have weight and food issues. Your parent or primary caregiver's responsiveness or sensitivity to your needs from infancy determines your personal attachment style. Babies attach to people who are sensitive and responsive in social interactions with them and who are consistently in their lives between ages six months and two years. As an infant learns to crawl and then walk, he uses his parents and other familiar people in his life as a secure base from which to explore his environment, knowing if he runs into any problems, he can return to that secure base for comfort and safety (Waters and Cummings 2000). You will learn more about attachment styles in the next chapter. For now, you would know that you had a secure attachment style as a child (and perhaps now) if you felt safe to engage with strangers, were upset when your mother left you, and were happy when she returned. You would also have felt as if your world was a safe place for you to explore and know that if you needed help, you could turn to your mother or primary caregiver.

Secure infants learn to trust their feelings, and they also learn to trust their view of the world, which originates from their parents or caregivers. Part of the emotional development of secure infants is learning to describe and communicate their emotions. Secure children spend more time expressing physical and emotional needs than do children who have been maltreated. If you experienced any of the childhood experiences mentioned in the above section, you may find it very difficult to regulate your feelings.

You may have also experienced emotions differently from the rest of your family, and this could also affect your attachment style (De Schipper, Oosterman, and Schuengel 2012). For example, sometimes parents who are very outgoing may encourage a shy child to be more socially interactive than she feels comfortable with, where a more sensitive parent would be more reassuring and supportive. Even without messages from the family, children who are more inhibited may develop ways to manage fear or anxiety that can later lead to overeating. Over time, for example, a shy child may continue to remove herself from social situations and turn to bingeing or overeating, leading to weight issues, depression, and anxiety (which exacerbate overeating) in later years. A family environment where there is a mismatch between the environment and the child's temperament, where a child's emotions are not validated by her parents or caregivers, or where emotional expressions are either ignored or invalidated can set the child up for later weight and eating problems. If you grew up in such a family, you learned to think that your view and experience of emotions is incorrect (Linehan 1993). This then may have caused you to have problems with emotional regulation because you never learned to identify, express, and regulate your emotions appropriately. This is very pertinent to your later problems with food and eating as most individuals with eating disorders (including binge-eating disorder) say that they have difficulty tolerating strong emotions and use food to avoid feeling or triggering such strong emotions or will use impulsive behaviors to manage them (Corstorphine et al. 2007; Van der Kolk and Fisler 1994).

If you grew up in a home where you learned that it is not acceptable or safe to express emotions, especially negative ones, this could have an effect on your eating behaviors in several ways: (1) you may have learned to "block" your awareness of these "unacceptable" or invalidated emotions through binge eating, purging (self-induced vomiting), or self-harming behaviors, or (2) you may have learned to block emotions through compulsive overeating, compulsive exercise, or restricting your food intake (Mountford et al. 2007; Waller, Kennerley, and Ohanian 2007). Individuals who were raised in a family where their parents invalidated their views or feelings are more likely to binge and purge or have other disordered eating behaviors. If your family put a lot of emphasis on achievement and success and the need to control one's emotions, you may have used compulsive exercise as a way of regulating your emotions (Haslam et al. 2008). Growing up in an invalidating environment could also be considered another childhood experience that causes toxic stress.

In the exercises below, see if you relate to any of the experiences either in childhood or adulthood, which can lead to problems with attachment (insecure attachment). In the next chapter, you will learn more about how these experiences can lead to specific attachment styles and how they can affect your weight and body image.

EXERCISE: **Traumatic Childhood Experiences**

Checkmark the traumatic childhood experiences you were exposed to before the age of eighteen.

☐ Were you often put down or insulted, or did you fear you would be physically hurt?

☐ Were your feelings invalidated or constantly questioned in your home? Were you told that what you felt did not matter?

☐ Did you have a parent or caregiver who constantly criticized you?

☐ Were you frequently physically abused (grabbed, shoved, slapped, or hit so hard you had bruises or injuries)?

☐ Did you feel as if your feelings were not accepted in your family?

☐ Did you feel that you were very different from your family members in terms of your feelings or any other ways?

☐ Were you sexually abused or touched inappropriately or forced to have sexual intercourse or to perform other sexual acts against your will?

☐ Did you live with someone who was an alcoholic or drug addict?

☐ Did anyone in your house suffer from a mental illness or attempt or commit suicide?

☐ Did you have a parent with a chronic illness?

☐ Did you have a parent with depression or anxiety that required hospitalization or in any way affected his or her ability to parent you?

☐ Did you feel as if your emotional needs were not met growing up?

☐ Was your mother or stepmother the victim of domestic violence?

☐ Did you witness violent acts that did not include your family (for example, someone was killed in front of you)?

☐ Were you bullied in school or at home?

☐ Did you ever feel that your emotions were not as important as your achievements?

☐ Did anyone you lived with go to jail?

If you have experienced any of the above childhood experiences, this may explain why you have difficulty regulating your emotions and why you may use food or other behaviors to try to control your emotions. These toxic childhood experiences often require specific treatment. Getting help from a therapist or counselor may help remove blocks caused by your traumas that keep you stuck using food for emotional regulation. Later chapters in this book will also help you begin to address these blocks and the toxic stress they caused.

EXERCISE: Traumatic Adult Experiences

Checkmark the experiences that happened to you after age eighteen.

☐ rape

☐ assault

☐ exposure to a life-threatening situation

☐ exposure to hurricane, tornado, or other natural disaster

☐ domestic violence

☐ abusive relationship

☐ death or serious illness of a loved one

☐ war or combat

☐ motor vehicle accident or plane crash

☐ exposure to a violent crime, such as a robbery or shooting

☐ other: _____

☐ other: _____

If you are like many of the people I work with who have food, body image, and weight problems, you have experienced numerous toxic childhood or adult experiences in your life. Remembering these difficult times may bring up a lot of emotions that you haven't felt in a long time. One way of thinking of these past experiences is to view yourself as the survivor that you are. Your spirit, or your soul, was strong enough to get you to this point in life. Later chapters in this book will enable you to recognize how healing will bring your strong, resilient soul the satisfaction it needs and the new life you deserve.

Whether you have a history of specific trauma, abuse, or neglect or you are just "wired differently" in terms of how strongly you feel your emotions and your ability to regulate your emotions, it is important to understand that emotions are often the driving forces behind your behaviors. If you focus on one without addressing the other, any changes you make will be temporary at best. Remember, weight problems are not about food; they are about how you use food. When you start to accept and honor your emotions and learn to regulate them without food, you will be able to address your soul's hunger, which is not for food but for self-expression and for healing. Later in this book, you will learn new skills for regulating your emotions so you don't have to use food to control, suppress, or numb your feelings.

CHAPTER 3

Embracing the Wisdom of the Body

Marla has difficulty expressing anger or fear and often completely disconnects from any sensations in her body associated with her emotions. She knows that she needs to be in touch with her body sensations to recognize when and if she is hungry or full, to recognize how food she eats affects her physically, and to identify and manage her emotions more effectively. Her dissatisfaction with her body started when she was very young, somewhere around age eight when her mother got sick and was in bed a lot of the time. Marla began to have to take care of her mother and her younger sister. Every day after school, she would find food for her sister and mother, help her sister with her homework, and get her to bed. Her mother wouldn't get out of bed for days, so sometimes there was little to eat in the house except crackers and peanut butter. Marla later found out that her mother wasn't sick; she was addicted to prescription pain pills. Her "bed days" were really the days she didn't have the money to buy her drugs and was going through withdrawal. During these times she was irritable and angry and often screamed at Marla and her sister to "just leave me alone." Then at other times, she was more loving and tried to be the mother Marla remembered from "before." Her mother also talked a lot about how fat she was and how much she hated her body. Marla often felt as if she was the only person holding her family together, and it was all she could do to get everything done each day and then fall into bed exhausted. She didn't have playdates with her friends because she just didn't have time to play. She couldn't remember a time in her life when she was aware of what she was feeling and how those emotions felt in the body. All she remembers is feeling unhappy with her body and feeling betrayed by her body for being bigger than she wants it to be.

If you've been struggling with your weight for most of your life, you may view your body as an adversary, as Marla does, when in fact it's your greatest ally. The body is the early warning system that helps you identify the emotions that are driving your behaviors. Your body can provide you with expert advice on what to eat and how much to eat. You can also use your body to experience true mindfulness by connecting to your body's wisdom and using your body to ground yourself emotionally.

When you experience negative feelings about your body, it may be the result of past hurtful experiences from childhood, which can lead to a disconnection between you and your body. This can lead to your self-evaluation (how you feel about yourself) being tied to your body size or shape, resulting in the use of unhealthy ways to lose weight or whip your body into shape. What most people don't know is that *your body is the reservoir of all the wisdom you need to change your life*. By changing your relationship with your body, you will be able to tap into its wisdom to heal. Use the exercise below to begin restoring your connection to your body and its sensations. This might be called a mindfulness exercise, but I like to call it a "mindless" exercise to point you in the direction of tapping into your body's wisdom rather than trying to use your intellect (mind) to figure things out or overthinking things. Repeat this exercise before you start any of the later exercises in this chapter so you can respond from a place of wisdom deep inside your body, connecting to your true or authentic self.

EXERCISE: **Mindful Mindlessness**

Sit in a comfortable chair with your feet flat on the floor. Be sure your back is well supported and that you are in a place where you will not be disturbed. This exercise is about reconnecting with your body, so just allow any thoughts you have to pass through your busy, active mind like leaves on a stream. Take three deep breaths. With the next breath, imagine your breath filling up your body completely from the top of your head to the tips of your toes. Then exhale, and allow all the air to be collected from all over your body and released in your exhalation. Now, imagine directing your breath to one part of your body at a time. As you do so, notice if any feelings or unwanted judgments come up for you, and then release them in your out-breath. Feel your breath first move into your scalp, your eyes, your face and jaw, your tongue, and the back of your neck; then exhale. Now move your breath into the front of your neck, into your throat, into your shoulders and out your arms, into your hands, and into the tips of your fingers; then exhale. Next move your breath into your upper chest and back, down into your belly and lower back, moving into and between your ribs and all your internal organs; then exhale. Finally, move your breath into your hips and belly, thighs and knees, then down your shins and calves and into your feet and toes; then exhale. Now, stop and take a moment to notice what your body feels like on the inside now that you have breathed the energy of your breath into it. Is it tingling? Are there different temperature sensations? Does it feel light or heavy? Does your body feel relaxed or tight? When was the last time you paid this much attention to the different parts of your body? Write your impressions below.

_____

_____

_____

_____

_____

_____

Stay with your body sensations as you read the rest of this chapter. If you find yourself drifting into your mind, just *gently* return your attention to breathing into your body and noticing what that feels like. Do this with kindness toward your body and without judgment.

What Is Body Image?

Body image is the picture you hold in your mind of your body. When you hold a negative picture or are dissatisfied with your body, it can be a significant predictor of compulsive overeating, binge eating, emotional distress, depression, problems in your relationships, or the use of steroids in men (Kanayama et al. 2006; Stice and Whitenton 2002). Having positive feelings about your body if you are in a bigger body may be difficult in a culture filled with images of the thin "ideal," but it's not impossible. Despite the overload of media images promoting thinness, a surprising number of media images are coming to the forefront of women and men in larger bodies who are refreshingly and courageously being themselves without regard to their body size. In 2012, *Seventeen* magazine signed the Body Peace Treaty, promising to "never change girls' body or face shapes in photos" after a petition started by an eighth-grader against airbrushed images in the magazine got over eighty thousand signatures (Hu 2012). In 2012, NOW (National Organization for Women) foundation celebrated the fifteenth birthday of Love Your Body Day. In the past year, thirty-five years after the publication of *Fat Is a Feminist Issue*, women and men who are living in larger bodies are stepping out of the shadows and proclaiming their desire to not make their lives about dieting and to not be less productive because of their size. The grassroots Health at Every Size movement is a big part of the attempt to turn around negative body image along with challenging the research studies that say fat is unhealthy (Bacon 2008).

These healthier images of people in larger bodies are important because they show that smaller size is not a prerequisite to being all you can be. When the media begins to portray people of all sizes and not just stereotype them in roles that diminish their essence or spirit (for example, fat people as comic figures in sitcoms), then it allows all of us to be the most that we can be—whatever that is for you as an individual, not as a number on the scale. The most important use of your body is not as a defining and limiting identity, but rather as the source of wisdom, no matter what size you are. Whenever you use your body size or shape to keep you from being who you want to be or who you truly are, you are stuck in fear. Being in fear and succumbing to its limits is a way of keeping yourself small. In the exercises below, take a look at how weight, size, and shape have influenced who you consider yourself to be (defined your identity) and ask yourself if this is the way you would like to continue to define yourself or if there is a greater, more important truth you want to live from.

EXERCISE: **Body Identity**

See if one or more of the identities listed below fit for you. Think of your body identity as a role or archetype you have chosen to play in your life for the time being until you are able and willing to be your best self. This is the way you've learned to cope with being in a bigger body. An archetype is a pattern that exemplifies a certain behavior or identity. See if you can use your body wisdom (keep breathing) to determine the truth underlying the role you play with your current body.

Sexy Mama Archetype: You are proud of your curves and feel you have a right to flaunt them. You may show off your body in tight-fitting clothing. Your sexiness may be misunderstood because what you really want is a stable relationship.

Truth: *I want to be loved for who I am.*

Truth: *When I'm acting sexy (even when it's not appropriate), what I really want is:*

_____

_____

Radical Archetype: You want to flip off anyone who calls you fat. Being angry is your way of coping with fat-shaming. You see yourself as a fierce fat activist.

Truth: *I want people to pay attention to me, and I want my voice to be heard.*

Truth: *If my anger could talk, it would say that what I really want is:*

_____

_____

Good Girl or Good Boy Archetype: You are a people-pleaser. You prefer to avoid conflict and want others to like you.

Truth: *I want to be accepted for who I am.*

Truth: *When I'm saying yes even when I want to say no, what I really want or need is:*

_____

_____

Do-Gooder Archetype: You are the person who can't say no. Sometimes people take advantage of you, but you don't mind because you're all about helping others.

Truth: *I want to be included, to be part of a group, team, or community.*

Truth: *If I could never help another person, what would be missing for me is:*

_____

_____

Power Broker Archetype: You like being in charge and running the show. You don't want to be perceived as weak or incapable.

Truth: *I want to be taken seriously in my career and in other areas of my life. I am strong and competent.*

Truth: *When I'm in charge, I feel:*

_____

_____

Big Mama: You see yourself as nurturing and nonthreatening. Your kid's friends like to come to your house, and you're the first one to bring goods for the bake sale. You feel guilty taking care of yourself.

Truth: *I want to know that I am worth caring for myself.*

Truth: *By taking care of other people, what I get for myself is:*

_____

_____

The Joker Archetype: You deflect any compliments or defuse conflict with humor. Everyone loves to be around you because you're "so funny."

Truth: *I want companionship. I don't want to be lonely.*

Truth: *Being funny helps me feel:*

_____

_____

Wounded Child Archetype: You feel as if life is against you and nothing will ever go your way.

Truth: *I want to be able to take care of myself and stand on my own two feet. I want others to see me as competent even when I don't always feel that way. All I need is a little support.*

Truth: *When I feel as if life is against me, what would help me feel stronger is:*

_____

_____

Big Man or Big Woman Archetype: You see yourself as someone who is naturally large and take on the role of the protector, the provider, or the strong man or woman. You believe in taking care of your family over all else.

Truth: *I want to be respected.*

Truth: *Being "large and in charge" keeps me from feeling:*

_____

_____

Other Body Identity: _____

Truth: _____

_____

_____

We all play many different roles in our lives or express different archetypes. These roles may be thrust on us by our parents, chosen unconsciously, or adopted with full awareness. For example, you may have been thrust into the Big Mama archetype by having to care-take your parents as child and then chosen to become a nurse or doctor (the Do-Gooder archetype) as Marla did. There is no right or wrong about the archetypes we exhibit in our lives. Having said that, it is good to be aware of these archetypes and how body size or shape may have unconsciously shaped our choices.

EXERCISE: **Role-Play**

Describe how your weight and food issues led you to play certain roles in your life, to choose certain careers, or even to marry or have relationships with certain people.

(Example: As a kid, I was bullied about my weight. This led to my desire to protect other kids who were teased. I am a teacher, and I love my work. I also have a firm stand in my classroom against bullying. My lack of self-confidence, however, led me to marry the first person who showed any interest in me, and it wasn't a good match for me.

My weight and food issues have shaped the roles I play in my life in the following ways...)

_____

_____

_____

_____

_____

_____

The next part of this exercise is about remembering who you are at your essence and recapturing the dreams you may have lost or thrown away because of limits you or others placed on you because of your body size. Before you begin, remember to take three deep breaths and reconnect with your body sensations. Imagine your body floating through air like a balloon—free and clear to move about wherever it wants to go. You can imagine your body floating on a cloud or floating into space. Experience the sensation of your body being free, not constrained by gravity or by the gravity of others' or your own expectations. With that feeling and staying in connection with your body sensations, describe the dreams you want to remember and bring back into your life.

(Example: I want to take ballet lessons.)

_____

_____

_____

_____

What are the needs (from archetypes above) that you want to find new ways to satisfy in your life?

_____

_____

_____

_____

Hopefully you are beginning to feel your way back to a relationship with your body. In the next section, you will learn more about the notion that the body stores your past experiences and about attachment styles (which were mentioned in chapter 2), and how these can affect how you feel about your body.

Parental Relationships and Body Image

Earlier, I discussed how the media and Western culture emphasize a certain ideal body size. Have you ever wondered why some people are more affected by these media images than others? Research is now showing that "attachment styles," which you learned about in the last chapter, may explain why (Cash, Theriault, and Annis 2004; Pace, Cacioppo, and Schimmenti 2012; Troisi et al. 2006). As you learned in the last chapter, a parent or caregiver's relationship with his or her child has a direct effect on the child's later social development, individual perceptions, emotions, thoughts, and expectations in future relationships. As it turns out, this pivotal early relationship also has an effect on the child's body image.

You learned about some of the childhood and adult experiences that can lead to unhealthy attachment in the last chapter. Those experiences create specific attachment styles. The connection between weight and body image issues has a lot to do with these attachment styles and whether they are secure (healthy) or insecure, as was the case with Marla.

If you got the message that adults are not reliable and that you should not trust people very easily, you may have developed one of several different insecure attachment styles. The list below shows the three most common insecure attachment styles, along with the parent behavior that can lead to that attachment style and its effect on the child and later on adult behavior and body esteem (Ainsworth et al. 1978; Benoit 2004; Main and Solomon 1986; Siegel 2013).

1. If your parents did not respond when you were upset or distressed as a child or if they discouraged crying and encouraged you to not lean on them for help, you may have developed *avoidant attachment*. If you've ever observed a child with avoidant attachment, she doesn't respond when the parent leaves and doesn't feel relieved when the parent returns. Children with avoidant attachment were treated as if they didn't need help when, in fact, they did. They grow up in an "emotional desert." If you had this experience as a child, you may be someone who has trouble even remembering your childhood. As an adult, you may experience problems in intimate relationships, feel disconnected from other people, and invest very little in your relationships. You may consider yourself to be "very independent" and tend to suppress your emotions. In the same way that you are avoidant in other relationships, you may also be disconnected from your body and have difficulty getting in touch with your body sensations associated with your emotions. You may be able to ignore body cues for hunger or fullness as well, leading to overeating and weight gain.

2. You may have developed an *ambivalent attachment* style if your parent or caregiver was very inconsistent—sometimes responsive, other times neglectful. You may have had to escalate your demands or act out to get your needs met. When your parents left even for short periods, you may have been distressed and angry and then had trouble warming up to them when they returned. You grew up in what is called an "emotional fog." As an adult, you may be perceived as less competent than you really are. People may annoyingly offer you help when you don't need or ask for it. You may feel that relationships are too stressful and too emotional, and you may frequently worry that your partner doesn't love you. When a relationship

ends, you may feel distraught. For you, emotions and body sensations may feel overwhelming, and you may use food to help you block or numb these feelings. For this reason, food can seem very comforting as it can be soothing when you feel distressed. This can lead to emotional overeating and weight gain.

3. A *disorganized attachment* style results from having a parent who exhibits frightening behavior or a parent who expects you, the child, to take care of the parent. It can also result from having parents who abuse or neglect you. If this was the situation you faced, you may have been afraid of your caregiver and have been confused as to how to get close to him or her. You may have grown up feeling disconnected from your emotions, or you may have dissociated from strong or overwhelming emotions. As an adult, you may suffer from symptoms of post-traumatic stress disorder or have unresolved trauma or loss issues. Memories and body sensations associated with your past traumas may feel as if they are happening right now, not in the past. Your body sensations and emotions may trigger flashbacks of trauma and loss and lead you to dissociate. If you dissociate, you basically feel detached from your immediate surroundings and your physical or emotional experience. This can feel as if you're watching a situation from outside of yourself and feeling you have no control over it, or you may have a moment where you feel as if the world is not real or appears flat and without emotional coloring. Sometimes when dissociation occurs, as during a traumatic experience, the person will not be able to remember what happened to him for hours or even years afterward. This can leave the person feeling easily stressed and overwhelmed, which can lead to stress eating. If you dissociate, you may also have had the experience of eating a box of donuts without even noticing that you were doing it because you were in a dissociated state. You may also feel very disconnected from your body.

If none of these scenarios fit for you, remember that almost 65 percent of children have secure, or healthy, attachment styles. Attachment problems in childhood don't mean you will definitely have problems in adulthood, but they do increase the risk. If you do have one of the insecure attachment styles, it can predispose you to destructive coping mechanisms, such as bingeing or compulsive overeating, and also to negative self-esteem and body image dissatisfaction (Cash, Theriault, and Annis 2004; McKinley and Randa 2005). Insecure attachment styles also can make you more sensitive to or overwhelmed by stress because the toxic stress associated with past traumas tends to put you on red alert (which is called hyperactive stress response; Fox and Hane 2008).

Insecure attachment doesn't just affect your stress response and how you handle emotions and body sensations, it can actually change how the nerve connections in your brain develop, and in cases of extreme neglect or trauma, can affect brain size (Insel and Young 2001; Perry 2009). Fortunately, the brain has plasticity, the ability to change and heal over time. So do you. If you become more aware of your attachment style, you can modify your responses to childhood experiences, heal past traumas or losses, and become more secure in your personal and romantic relationships.

Attachment styles are also shaped by our personality and genetics. For example, you may have had a very supportive family growing up, but you may have naturally been more anxious and insecure from birth. Your personality traits may have influenced how you responded to your family dynamics and your relationship with your parent or primary caregiver (Belsky and Rovine 1998; Gillath et al. 2008).

Attachment Styles and Body Image

Just as romantic and friendship relationships are affected by the early relationship with your primary caregiver, your relationship with your body is also affected. People who didn't receive nurturing as an infant may not be able to nurture themselves as adults. If you tend not to trust others, you may view your body with mistrust. For example, when you sense a body sensation related to an emotion or just a simple body cue of hunger, you may second-guess that message from your body. If you have difficulty connecting emotionally with others, you may also have trouble feeling a sense of compassion or connection to your body. What's important is to identify ways in which your early attachment relationships have affected your relationship with your body and ways to make needed changes.

EXERCISE: Your Caregiver Relationship Story

Write a short story of your early relationship with your primary caregiver. Describe how that relationship has had an effect on your life. (Example: *I realized from the chart above that I have an avoidant personality style, and this explains why I've had so much trouble in my relationships. Now I see that it's not something wrong with me; it's a pattern that I've been operating from without even knowing it. I thought I was just really independent and that men couldn't deal with that. But I can see now that my trust issues come from my relationship with my mother, who was not very emotionally available.*)

_____

_____

_____

_____

_____

_____

_____

_____

_____

Now go back over your story above to see if you can identify your attachment style by the narrative. For example, does your story have mostly emotional content? If so, you are more likely to have an ambivalent attachment style. If your story is very logical and almost devoid of emotions, you may fit more with the avoidant attachment style. If you reread your story and find it very disconnected, going from past to future, or "all over the place," you may have a disorganized style. In the space below, see if you can rewrite your story in a more balanced way—adding in emotional content where appropriate, keeping the narrative more linear (from start to finish), or making it more logical if it is too emotional (by stating the facts). This is a way to start using the parts of your brain that may be underdeveloped because of your early childhood relationships with your parent or caregiver. This integration process is part of what you need to move toward more secure attachment.

_____

_____

_____

_____

_____

_____

_____

_____

_____

In the space below, describe how your early attachment relationship may have affected how you felt about your body. (*Example: I never trusted anyone in my life. In every relationship, I always expected to be left. I never thought I could trust anyone to take care of me. This is the same with my body. I don't trust my body at all. I'm always second-guessing my feelings and doubting my body sensations. Do I really feel angry, or am I just exaggerating? I look at my body as just another person [or thing] that has let me down and disappointed me because it's not the way it should be [thin].*)

_____

_____

_____

_____

_____

_____

_____

A free online test can help you determine your specific attachment style: http://www .yourpersonality.net. You can also see how your attachment style shows up in romantic relationships by taking a different version of the test at http://personality-testing.info/tests /ECR.php. Later in this chapter, I will discuss ways in which you can move toward a more secure attachment style in your relationship with your body.

Remember, you should speak with a therapist or psychologist if you feel you need support or treatment for childhood trauma, abuse, or neglect.

Body Sensations and Having a Mindful Relationship with Food

As one of my teachers (Ghazaleh Lowe from Academy of Intuition Medicine) once said, "The body is always in the present moment—it has no other choice." Think about this for a moment. While the mind is always flitting away from what's happening now to what might happen in the future, the body is steadfastly staying with, enduring, and processing the present. For example, if you're struggling with memories or thoughts from your past, such as, *My mother favored my brother over me*, you can check in with your body sensations to see if you are (1) the adult reflecting on the past to gain insight and to heal or (2) your child self who is continually reliving past hurts like a reel of film that is on repeat. One way to know if you are in your child self is that the emotions may seem much stronger than they logically should. Or you may notice yourself using a younger person's way of speaking. For example, in a conversation with one of my clients about his concern about his mother dating a much younger woman, I asked him how he felt about this. He responded by making a face of disgust and said, "Yuck." "Yuck" was a term his eleven-year-old self used, not one his thirty-five-year-old self would use. Usually when you are in your child self, there's also a feeling of helplessness—you feel unable to do anything to change the situation. This is generally a more common experience for a child than for a competent adult. The experience is often one that has come up before—something you have a difficult time resolving or letting go of.

What's the difference? If you are grounded in the present moment, you will be able to feel body sensations and emotions pass through you and you will metabolize your experience in the moment. While the experience you are processing may be painful, you will feel your body release the pain bit by bit, allowing you to return to your life in the present moment, feeling a sense of completion. We all know that feeling. For example, when you suffer the loss of a loved one, you may cry at the time, and then over a period of sometimes years, your grief may be triggered and you may find sadness, anger, or other emotions well up from deep within (your body's memories). When you allow yourself to feel those emotions in the moment, they pass with time. When, however, you block your emotions with food or with other behaviors, you judge what happened ("That shouldn't have happened"), or you judge how you feel ("I should be over this by now"), the emotions continue to stay in storage in your body, triggering your defense mechanisms to help you cope—overeating, bingeing, numbing yourself, and so on.

If you check in with your body when you are upset about something, ask yourself, *How old do I feel right now?* and realize you are experiencing a situation from the point of view of your child self, you know you are not in the present moment. You are either in the past or fearing that something from the past will affect your future. You can confirm this by checking in with your body sensations. When you are thrown into the past, with memories of an old hurt, you will be "in your head"—in your mind rehashing old hurts—having lots of judgments and emotions, and it will be difficult to connect to the body. Grounding yourself in the present moment will enable you to gain more insight into your situation, and you do this by focusing on the feelings and sensations in your body, allowing the mind to do what it does while you put your attention on your body sensations. In the exercise below, you will have an opportunity to practice this.

EXERCISE: **Processing Old Stories**

Write down a situation from your past that continues to bother you. It could be something small, or it could be something very significant. Describe your emotions, body sensations, thoughts, and judgments. Write how it made you feel about yourself. Remember to balance your story as described in a previous exercise based on your attachment style. If you tend to be coldly logical, add in more right-brain emotionality. If you tend toward being overly emotional, see if you can use more of your left-brain logic. Try to write the story in a cohesive fashion, with a beginning, middle, and end. Don't get lost in the details.

_____

_____

_____

_____

_____

Next, while sitting in a comfortable chair, begin to pay attention to your breathing. Close your eyes if you feel comfortable doing so. If not, just find a point of focus in the room and put your attention on that. Then, simply notice the air moving into your nostrils and feel it moving out with your out-breath. Continue for three full breaths. Next, imagine your breath moving throughout your body from the top of your scalp to the bottoms of your feet. Notice the sensation or energy of your breath moving through your body. Feel the sensation in your nose and throat. Feel your breath expanding your lungs and then moving down your arms. Notice any tingling or warmth in your hands. Now feel your breath moving into your belly and down your back, down your legs, and into your feet. Put your attention now on the inner sensations of your feet. Do this for three more breaths, keeping your attention on the sensations in your feet. When you are ready, bring your attention back to the present moment, noticing your feet flat on the floor, and then slowly and gently open your eyes.

Now go back and reread your story above. Then answer the questions below.

1. How old was the person who wrote this story (based on language, sentiment, and insight)? _____

2. What are the *facts* of the story? (What are the actual events that anyone reading this would agree on? This does not include your emotions or judgments, which are based on your perceptions.) See if you can take a bird's-eye view or observer position and look at your story as if someone else wrote it.

   _____

   _____

   _____

3. List below all the judgments, opinions, and emotions found in the story.

   _____

   _____

   _____

   _____

   _____

4. Taking a few more deep breaths and, feeling the sensations in your feet and throughout your body, see if you can identify why you are holding on to this hurt from your past. I've listed a few reasons that clients have shared with me about similar situations to help you get started.

    • If I let this go, then I feel I will be losing the memory of the person I lost.

    • I feel that holding on to this memory or situation will keep me from making the same mistake in the future.

    • I'm holding on because I'm getting something out of it (feeling loved, feeling needed, feeling as if I matter).

    • _____

    _____

    _____

Reminding yourself to keep your attention on your breath moving in and out of your nostrils and to focus on the sensations in your feet, ask yourself if you feel ready to let this hurt from the past go—at least in this moment. If the answer is yes, list one ritual you will do right now to let go. I've listed some ideas that might help.

• I will find a token to represent my memory of the loved one I lost (crystal, candle, picture, other), and I will make a home altar where every morning I will sit in silence for several minutes. I will do this for one month to honor my loved one.

• I will write down the situation and then bury the paper under a tree in the park (or burn the paper and bury the ashes).

• I will call a friend I trust and ask him or her to support me by reminding me of my desire to let this past hurt go. We will discuss what would be the appropriate reminder.

• I will make an appointment with my therapist to discuss this issue with the intention of working my way to forgiveness, letting go, and releasing the pain.

My ritual: _____

_____

_____

_____

As you can see from this exercise, holding on to the past not only affects your perception of your current circumstances and triggers emotions that may lead to overeating or bingeing, but also keeps you from enjoying your life in each moment now. At the end of your life, what would have served you most—living the life you have now or holding on to the life you lived in the past? The present is the only thing we can really have any effect on. We can't change the past no matter how hard we try. We can heal the past, but only by being in the present moment and being in our bodies (not in our intellect alone— judging, reliving past pain, and creating suffering). In the upcoming sections of this chapter, you will learn how you may have come to experience disconnection with your body, how mindfulness can help you change your relationship with your body, and how to use your body sensations and body wisdom to live more fully.

Body Disconnection and Obsession: Two Sides of the Same Coin

Sometimes dissatisfaction with your body may cause you to disconnect from it—ignoring body cues, looking only at your face in the mirror, avoiding looking in mirrors altogether, or avoiding tight clothing to avoid addressing feelings of discomfort about body shape or size. This also disconnects you from your body sensations and, most importantly, from the wisdom your body has to offer. If you think about it, disconnection from your body may make your attempts to whip your body into shape with excessive or extreme exercise or with painfully restrictive diets easier, but it will make it more difficult for you to maintain a healthy weight and to enjoy eating and moving.

Another way in which body disconnection shows up is as an excessive preoccupation with the body through body checking—pinching parts of the body to check for fatness. In fact, you may be one of the over 50 percent of individuals with binge-eating disorder (BED) who engage in regular body checking (Reas et al. 2005). Yet another example of how you may obsess about or avoid your body is through either obsessive weighing or avoiding the scale altogether. As you can see in the above discussion, attachment styles can also affect how you connect with body sensations associated with emotions.

EXERCISE: Tapping into Body Wisdom

Now, take three deep breaths, allow your body to relax, and put your feet flat on the floor. Imagine the bottoms of your feet are reaching down to the center of the earth, grounding you and calming you. Let go of distracting thoughts, and allow your body to feel as if it is sinking into the chair and directly grounded to the center of the earth. Remember that your body always speaks in kindness, not in negativity. Your body only wants you to know love, not pain. With that in mind, answer the questions below.

1. If you were to listen to your body's wisdom, how would you address your negative body thoughts differently? (*Example: I would interrupt these negative thoughts and speak more kindly to my body.*)

   _____

   _____

   _____

2. If you were to listen to your body's wisdom, what would it say to you about your current size and shape? (*Example: My body knows that I am committed to improving my health and fitness. I'm on a journey to healing that will benefit my body, mind, and spirit.*)

   _____

   _____

   _____

Trauma and Your Relationship with Your Body

Bessel van der Kolk, a noted post-traumatic stress disorder (PTSD) expert, has shown that trauma has a direct effect on the body, causing it to be frozen in a state of fear or on red alert (hypervigilant). He says: "What most people do not realize is that trauma is not the story of something awful that happened in the past, but the residue of imprints left behind in people's sensory and hormonal systems" (Integral Yoga Magazine 2009, 12). When you experience certain body sensations, certain smells, certain sounds, being touched in a certain way, or even the texture or smell of certain foods that trigger your trauma memories, you may feel terrified, as though the trauma is happening to you right now (Integral Yoga Magazine 2009; Van der Kolk 1994; Van der Kolk 2005). Van der Kolk (1994) proposed that "the body keeps the score" in response to trauma. Traumatic experiences are stored in what is called "body memory" as opposed to conscious memory. You may have experienced this phenomenon, which may have made it difficult for you to remember or talk about your past trauma.

Trauma also triggers the stress response (fight-flight-freeze), causing you to feel as if you are constantly on red alert. This can make it difficult for you to regulate your emotions and soothe yourself during times of stress. And it may be one of the reasons you use food (or alcohol, drugs, sex, or gambling) to self-regulate, self-soothe, and deal with stress.

Eckhart Tolle, the well-known author and spiritual teacher, said: "Most humans are never fully present in the now, because unconsciously they believe that the next moment must be more important than this one. But then you miss your whole life, which is never not now" (Burkeman 2009). Healing also only happens in the present moment. We can't go back and change the past, and we have no way to predict or control the future. By staying in touch with your body, you can ground yourself in the present by refocusing on your body's sensations. The body is where you start to heal from past hurts, trauma, and abuse. The body is constantly offering you wise feedback on what to eat, when to eat, and how much to eat. (You will learn more about how to identify body cues about food in chapter 6.) Your body is your best friend. And despite what it has gone through, it has continued to work on your behalf throughout your lifetime. Listen to your body's eloquent voice, make your body your ally, and use your body to live in the present, moment by moment.

CHAPTER 4

Level Four: Creating New Core Beliefs

David and his older brother often got into fights over David's mother being more protective of David, her youngest child. He coped by finding comfort and solace in food. As a result he was overweight as a child. By the time he was a teenager, he was bigger than his brother, and unconsciously he felt safer and less vulnerable when he was bigger and heavier. When his brother tried to fight with him, David was no longer afraid. As an adult, he was able to identify a core belief from his past of "bigger is better," which explained his difficulty in staying at his desired weight.

Unconscious core beliefs can stand between you and your goal to put an end to your food, body image, and weight issues. When first formed, usually when you were younger and during times of transition, trauma, or emotional upheaval, core beliefs are solutions to problems you couldn't solve—perhaps because you didn't have the resources at the time. For example, you may have learned not to show any emotion as a child as a way to avoid being hurt, or because you believed that your intense emotions would hurt another person. Your core belief, in this case, might be "Showing others how I feel is dangerous." And this strategy can be detrimental in many areas of your adult life. Understanding that such damaging core beliefs no longer function for you will help you shift to new guiding principles that will serve you better.

Being Aware of Core Beliefs

For the purposes of our work together, core beliefs are beliefs that usually formed when you were younger and during times of trauma, transition, or emotional upheaval and later became unconscious. Core beliefs represent the way you see yourself, other people, the world, and your future. Core beliefs are usually related to primal needs, such as the need for safety, attention, recognition, love, and trust, and are activated in situations that you perceive as threatening to these primal needs. These beliefs were formed as a way of coping with some problem that perhaps you were too young or too inexperienced to deal with. If you received unwanted attention from boys because you developed earlier than your peers, for example, you may have formed the belief, *If I gain weight, I will be less attractive and will feel safer*, or *I'm not safe unless I'm in a bigger body*. Being overweight may have served the purpose of protecting you from this unwanted attention. However, this core belief, while it may have helped you cope in the past, now stands between you and a healthy relationship with your body and a healthy weight. The belief no longer serves the purpose it once did.

Negative core beliefs are more common in individuals with obesity and binge-eating disorder than in individuals without these issues. Research highlights the importance of addressing these negative core beliefs; when they are not addressed, you may find it more difficult to stop unhealthy behaviors (Leung, Waller, and Thomas 2000; Sines et al. 2008; Van Hanswijck et al. 2003; Waller 2003). Negative core beliefs play an important role in the development and maintenance of the symptoms of eating disorders and in weight gain (Unoka, Tolgyes, and Czobor 2007). Core beliefs have also been implicated in the difficulty some women with food and weight issues have in becoming more aware of and learning to express their emotions (Lawson et al. 2008). The presence of negative core beliefs can lead to compulsive behaviors, such as compulsive overeating, bingeing, purging, and restricting. Adverse parenting experiences in childhood are associated with disordered eating of all types including compulsive overeating and binge eating. It may be that children in these situations develop core beliefs as a way to avoid painful or frightening emotions, and that explains why adverse parenting leads, in some cases, to disordered eating (Sheffield et al. 2009).

Origination of Core Beliefs

Core beliefs come out of adverse childhood experiences or insecure attachment styles. Sometimes core beliefs are related to trauma, abuse, or neglect, but they can also originate from other experiences you had in your family growing up. Below is a list of some typical family scenarios that lead to specific beliefs (Young, Klosko, and Weishaar 2003). See if you can match your family situation with any core beliefs you may hold.

Children from explosive, detached, abusive, or unpredictable homes may have one (or more) of the following beliefs:

- I can't count on others to be there for me, and I will always lose the ones I love.

- Others will take advantage of me.

- I don't belong. I'm an outsider.

- Something is wrong with me, and no one will love me if they really get to know me.

- I haven't lived up to my potential, so why try?

Children with enmeshed (overly close) relationships with a parents, where their judgment is undermined or who come from overprotective homes, may develop one of these beliefs:

- I can't take care of myself. I feel incompetent.

- I don't feel safe in the world.

- I don't have any direction. I feel like I'm floundering in my life.

- I feel like a failure. I feel inadequate.

Children from permissive and overly indulgent homes don't learn to respect others and have poor internal limits and boundaries. Their core beliefs may be one of the following:

- I should be able to have or do whatever I want when I want.

- I get easily frustrated. I have a hard time controlling my impulses to do certain things.

Homes where children are taught to put aside their own needs and emotions to gain attention, approval, or love may develop these core beliefs:

- I feel my needs are not as important as pleasing others. I am afraid to express my emotions for fear someone will get angry or upset at me.

- I feel guilty if I put my needs before others'.

- Status, money, and achievement are very important to me.

Children who grow up in a home with too many rules learn to suppress, control, or ignore their feelings to avoid making mistakes or breaking the rules and may develop core beliefs such as:

- I believe that what can go wrong, will! I try my hardest not to make mistakes.

- I fear that my emotions will harm others or that I will be embarrassed or abandoned if I let people know how I feel.

- No matter what I do, it's never good enough.

- If people don't meet my expectations or I don't meet my own expectations, I feel they or I should be punished.

As discussed above, core beliefs may come from early childhood experiences or may be formed during periods of transition or upheaval in your life. Sometimes core beliefs can come from a perception you have about what someone else thinks about you or from a statement made by a family member or friend that, for whatever reason, stuck with you.

Another type of experience that can lead to the formation of negative core beliefs is childhood neglect. Childhood neglect is defined as the failure of a parent or caregiver to provide needed food, clothing, shelter, medical care, or supervision to the degree that the child's health, safety, and well-being are threatened with harm (Turney and Tanner 2005).

Parental neglect and physical abuse in childhood may be a more potent predictor of obesity than even sexual abuse, increasing your risk of being overweight by 50 percent (Bentley and Widom 2009; Lissau and Sorensen 1995; Temple University 2007).

Effects of Core Beliefs

Core beliefs represent patterns that are formed in childhood but then are repeated (usually unconsciously) over and over. You'll know you are in one of your core belief patterns because you'll have the same emotions, thoughts, judgments, body sensations, and behaviors every time you find yourself behaving from one of your primary core beliefs. You may repeat the pattern of childhood emotional abuse in a clear way by being in relationships with partners who are emotionally abusive. Or you may try to fight the pattern by doing just the opposite of what your belief tells you to do. For example, a person who feels inadequate and fears failure may work eighty hours a week in an attempt to avoid failure. Often the overworking will backfire, and she will get sick or become depressed and be unable to work, thereby increasing her sense of failure. Another way of maintaining a core belief is by trying to avoid it. For example, if you learned that you couldn't trust others to be there for you, you may avoid making friends and having intimate relationships. You may describe yourself as a "loner," when in fact you are just unconsciously acting from a core belief. These attempts only reinforce the mistrust belief because other people pick up on your distance or coldness and distance themselves from you. No matter how your core belief is being kept in place, when it is triggered, you will feel intense emotions, which can serve as a clue to the presence of a core belief that no longer serves you. These core beliefs can also underlie a persistent problem in your life—such as repeated failures at reaching and maintaining a healthy weight or recurrent binge eating. Almost always, it's a core belief that is in the way of achieving what you desire. Whatever your core belief, if it is in opposition to your current goals and desires, it will benefit you to identify this belief and decide to change it if it is no longer in your best interest.

In the exercise below, you will have an opportunity to identify core beliefs that you may be holding on to, perhaps unconsciously. You'll recognize your core belief because it's the niggling thought that may be in the back of your mind when something goes wrong. You can also recognize the presence of a core belief because it is usually associated with intense emotions. Sometimes you'll still feel intense emotion about a situation that happened a long time ago or that others feel you shouldn't be upset about. The core belief affects not only your relationship with food and your body but also your other relationships, how you handle stress, and your overall well-being.

EXERCISE: Identifying Your Core Belief

Find a quiet place where you can relax and work on this exercise without interruption.

1. Consider why you have struggled with your weight for so long. (*Example: I love to eat.*)

   _____

2. Ask yourself what would be missing in your life if your current behaviors around food were no longer an option. For example, what would be missing from your life if you had an accident resulting in a broken jaw and your jaw had to be wired? (I know it's extreme, but let's just pretend.)

   _____

   _____

3. If the above were true, what is your worst fear about what would happen? To get to the heart of that fear, write at least three statements in the following format: If (how I felt or what happened), then my biggest fear would be _____. Here are some questions you can ask yourself:

   a. If that happened, then what?

   b. If that's true, what does that mean?

   c. What does that say about me?

   d. What's my worst fear if that was true?

   Keep going through the questions until you get to a primal need, such as the need for safety, recognition, attention, acceptance, love, or companionship. (*Example: If I couldn't eat what I wanted, I'd feel like a weak person. If I were weak,*

I'd feel something was wrong with me. If something were wrong with me, I would feel unlovable.)

_____

_____

_____

4. If you had difficulty coming up with your core belief, look at the list below and see if any resonate with you, or go through the family situations (above) that are associated with core beliefs and choose one from there.

- What I want or need is not important to others (so I might as well go along with what they want to avoid problems).

- I'm better than other people, so why don't I have _____?

- I'm a failure. I am stupid. I am less successful than I should be.

- I feel empty. I'm floundering. I have no direction.

- I am incompetent. I can't take care of myself; I feel helpless.

- No one would love me if they really knew who I am, what I've done, or how I feel.

- I don't belong. I feel unwanted, isolated, or different from others.

- I am imperfect, or something is wrong with me.

- I am a bad or unworthy person. (If this is true for you, you may be hyper-sensitive to criticism or rejection.)

- I'm weak, and bad things will happen to me because of that.

- Other people will take advantage of me. I always get the short end of the stick; I often feel cheated.

- I don't feel safe.

- I can't depend on other people to meet my needs.

5. Write your core belief below. It is usually the combination of some part of your very first "if-then-fear" statement and your last. Using the example above, "If I am weak, then I am unlovable." So in this case, food represents love to you. Food is being used to fill a need for love that is not being met in other ways. Your fear of or judgments about being weak may include weakness around food, exercise, how you treat your body, relationships, or work, and they probably developed sometime during your childhood. Ask yourself where "being weak" or "fearing that I'm weak" (or your core belief) shows up in your life and how you cope with it.

_____

_____

_____

_____

6. Describe how areas of your life are affected by your core belief.

Financial success: _____

_____

Work/career: _____

_____

Eating: _____

_____

Body image: _____

_____

Love relationships: _____

_____

Friendships: _____

_____

Feelings of self-worth: _____

_____

Security, feeling safe: _____

_____

Feeling part of a group, belonging: _____

_____

Other: _____

_____

7. Describe a memory or time in your life that may be connected to or the start of your core belief. (Example: *I remember when I stayed with my grandmother when Mom was sick. I was really scared that something bad would happen to my mother. She said I had to "be strong" for my mother. Instead of understanding my fear, my grandmother spent a lot of time focusing on what I was eating. She wouldn't let me eat some of my favorite foods.*)

_____

_____

_____

_____

Are there any other insights you can draw from the way you currently use food and your memories from childhood? What other purpose does food serve in your life? How does food help you deal with emotions?

_____

_____

_____

_____

If you were abused or neglected as a child, you are a trauma survivor. If you feel your needs were not met for any reason in childhood, you may no longer recognize that your eating problems either started after these experiences or became worse after a traumatic experience. If that is the case, I strongly recommend that you work with a therapist specializing in trauma. Getting therapeutic help does not mean you will have to relive all of what happened to you. But trauma often lives in the body as well as in the mind and spirit. Therefore, simply losing weight will not solve your problem. In fact, losing weight may make your core belief pop up with a vengeance, which could lead to your regaining your weight.

Changing Your Core Beliefs

Being under the influence of core beliefs is like living in a dream. When you're asleep and you have a vivid dream, the dream seems completely real. You may feel as if what's happening in the dream is really happening. When you experience fear in a dream, for example, your heart rate may increase and you may even breathe more rapidly. But when you wake up, you are able to look back over the dream with a different point of view and recognize that the dream wasn't real. The same experience can occur when you identify a prominent core belief.

In order to change a core belief, you have to change your perspective (wake up from the dream). For example, David's belief that "bigger is better" affected his marriage. His wife was the financial "heavyweight" in the family, and David even worked for her family's business. In his marriage, when he would lose weight, he often felt too vulnerable, which led to him regaining the weight. At work, his insecurities also reinforced his need to be in a bigger body, to metaphorically be able to have more substance. His perspective that he was not safe, that he didn't have enough power unless he was bigger, was a child or teen's view of his life situation. When he became aware of this core belief and its effect on his adult life, he could shift his perspective and see the belief from an adult viewpoint. By identifying this core belief and recognizing that it came from his childhood experiences but wasn't really part of his current life experience, he could choose to change his belief to one that was more in line with his current goals. His desire was to be fit enough to do activities with his daughters. His new core belief was motivated by this desire: "When I take care of my body in a healthy way, I am able to do more things with my kids."

Another way core beliefs affect us is that we believe other people see us through the lens of the core belief we hold. For example, David believed that when he was thinner, his wife saw him as less powerful, more vulnerable. This part of core beliefs is based on myth alone and is part of what is called magical thinking of childhood. Children assume that everything is as they see it, and when you have a core belief originating in childhood, it may feel as if people are judging you or seeing you in the way you see or judge yourself. Or your belief itself may have been based on someone telling you that you are weak, you are stupid, or no one will love you if you're fat. Below is an exercise to help you shift your perception about your beliefs. While your child self may believe with all your heart that the belief is true or that what someone told you to believe is true, your mature self can counter that belief to show you it is not true all the time or ever.

EXERCISE: **Perception Shifting**

1. Has someone ever told you something about you that stuck with you or that led to one of your core beliefs? (*Example: My dad constantly called me Miss Piggy and told me I'd never get a man or even have friends if I were fat.*)

    _____

    _____

    _____

2. Now see if you can challenge that belief by providing evidence as if you were in a court of law arguing that the statement or belief above is *not* true. What experiences do you have that show this belief is not true all the time? (*Example: I have large friends who are happily married. I've been in relationships where I felt loved and valued even when I was heavy.*)

    _____

    _____

    _____

71

3. What steps would you be willing to take to challenge your core belief in real life? (*Example: I've decided to work with a therapist to reduce my fears of dating and having a relationship, and I'm really going to treat myself as I would like others to treat me.*)

_____

_____

_____

When you become aware of your core beliefs, you can decide to honor their place in your life and the earlier benefit you received. For example, David's belief, "Bigger is better," made him feel safe against his older brother. You can also recognize that you are no longer the frightened, sad, or rebellious child or teen who first developed this belief, and become aware of the fact that you have more skills for dealing with life's problems than you did as a child. Finally, now that you are an adult, your current needs and challenges may be different from those of your younger self, and therefore, your core beliefs may no longer apply. In the exercises below, you will be able to let go of old core beliefs and develop new guiding principles.

EXERCISE: **Letting Go of Core Beliefs**

1. How did your core belief serve you when it first developed?

_____

_____

_____

2. What skills do you have for getting your needs met that you didn't when you were younger? (*Example: I know how to analyze situations differently. I can distract myself when I feel overwhelmed.*)

_____

_____

_____

3. What would you say to your younger self to acknowledge him or her for doing the best he or she could do at the time your core belief was formed? *(Example: "I know you did your best. You aren't to blame for what happened.")*

_____

_____

_____

4. Are you ready to let that core belief go? Yes _____ No _____

5. If yes, write your new guiding principle below. For example: If your core belief was, "I'm not safe unless I'm in a bigger body," your guiding principle might be, "I depend on my adult skills to keep me safe as I focus on my health and well-being."

_____

_____

_____

6. If you answered no, write your reasons for holding on and the steps you can commit to taking to either (1) get clear on whether you should let this belief go or (2) understand and release pain from the past that keeps your belief stuck.

_____

_____

_____

If you've been able to let go of your old core belief(s), congratulations! If you are not quite ready to take that step, don't be too hard on yourself. You may want to mark your calendar to revisit this chapter in a month, three months, and six months to see if time and insight allow you to take this step. Knowing what you need to do, however, is not enough to actually keep a new change in place. You have to practice and use the new guiding principles you've developed in your everyday life so it becomes a permanent change, rather than a flash-in-the-pan insight that dissipates with time. In the next exercise, you can choose how you'd like to practice.

EXERCISE: **Practicing Your New Guiding Principles**

1. Choose one action you can take today to remind yourself of your new guiding principle. Here are some suggestions to get you started:

    a. List your guiding principle in your calendar with a daily alarm so you start your day remembering.

    b. Choose an object that symbolizes your new guiding principle (this could be a crystal, a plant, or a picture, for example) and keep it on your bedside table or your desk.

    c. Keep a list of the signs you are in your old pattern (emotions, body sensations, usual behaviors, and post-behavior emotions), and see if you can identify the pattern by journaling about any upsetting experiences you have in your day. Most of these upsetting experiences will lead you back to your pattern, and you can journal about skills you could use to break the pattern and reinforce your new guiding principle.

    d. Other ideas you have for practicing new guiding principles:

    _____

    _____

By completing this chapter, you have taken another difficult step toward freeing yourself from your weight, food, and body image issues. The "Body Appreciation Meditation," a guided audio meditation available at http://www.newharbinger.com/32127, is designed to help you tap into the wisdom of your body and shift your relationship with your body to a more positive one. In the next chapter, you will be able to reconnect with the part of yourself that was never changed by any of your life experiences. By doing so, you can draw on the strength of this part of yourself that is unchanging, ever present, and always "in your corner." From here, you will have the opportunity to start rewriting the parts of your life story that you choose to change and moving forward from strength, hope, and love (of yourself).

CHAPTER 5

Level Five: Finding Soul Satisfaction

Erica was successful in her work as an executive assistant and had accomplished many of her financial goals. However, during treatment for binge-eating disorder, she realized that her bingeing was driven by fear and anxiety, due in great part to her childhood. Her father was a larger-than-life person who did everything to extremes, including drinking in excess. When he was drunk, he was often violent or threatening to her mother and sometimes toward her. When she came home from school, she never knew what her evenings would be like. Would she feel safe or feel the need to hide in her room to avoid him? This insecurity followed her into adult life. Her fear was that she was not good enough to pursue the job she dreamed of as an ICU nurse. With ongoing therapy, she was able to recognize that the insecurity and fear that kept her from her dreams came from her childhood, and that now, as an adult, she was able to choose to live the life that she had dreamed of. By reconnecting to her unrealized passion, she found other areas of her life falling into place—including being able to stop bingeing and maintaining a healthy weight for the first time in her life.

In the past four chapters, you've learned how your behaviors, emotions, core beliefs, and body sensations relate to your struggles with food, your weight, and your body. Each of these previous levels has prepared you for what I will discuss in this chapter: how to reach soul satisfaction. At some point, you will come to realize that changing your appearance is no longer about matching Western culture's ideal of what you should look like; but rather, who you are on the inside and being able to express your true and authentic self, no matter what your size or shape, is what will lead to satisfaction. If you ask yourself what the cause is of most of your suffering about your weight, body dissatisfaction, and food issues, you may realize that it is because of these problems that you are not able to express who you truly are. In this chapter, you will learn how to do just that—find soul satisfaction and bring it into all areas of your life, including your relationship with food, how you feel about your body, and your weight.

What Is Soul Satisfaction?

The soul is the part of us that is unchanging and separate from the thoughts, judgments, and experiences of our day-to-day lives. This part of ourselves, our essence or our true self, is what makes us individuals because it is expressed differently in different people. No matter what you go through in life, this part of your self is the part of you that remains without change, unblemished, and not tarnished by life's tawdriness or pain. If you meditate, you may have experienced a sense of stillness, in which thoughts pass through without hooking you or disturbing your peacefulness. That stillness is one place where you can access your soul-self. If you've gone through a difficult period in your life, as I did after the death of my middle son, you may describe this part of yourself as what helped you get through that dark time. It's the "x factor" that gives you the energy to survive all of life's trials and tribulations and still maintain hope and sometimes optimism. It's that part of you that can restore the joy of living. Satisfying your soul is about living from who you truly are, being anchored by your essential nature. Soul satisfaction is the anchor that grounds you to the greater truth of who you are.

What Does It Mean to Be Anchored?

Being anchored is about being true to yourself and accessing your inner strength. Sometimes life's struggles can change you and take you off your path or make you lose your focus in life. When you find your true anchor in life, you tap into a vast reservoir of intuitive, natural knowledge that will help you shift your beliefs, use your body sensations and body wisdom as cues, regulate your emotions, and manage your behaviors. Without this deep well of knowledge in which body, mind, and soul are connected, you will continue to operate on superficial levels, repeating past mistakes, reenacting old traumas, and living your life based on beliefs that no longer serve you.

You may feel that your weight or troubling life experiences have typecast you in a life role that doesn't really suit you. When you are able to live more from your authentic self, you will feel like a storm-tossed sailor who has found a safe harbor in which to drop anchor. You will feel like you've come home—to your self. If you anchor to your authentic self, nothing can ever truly shake you. Finding your anchor may be about work or relationships or any area of your life in which you are not yet being fully authentic. When you find your anchor, you live from who you truly are, and as a result, your relationship with food and your body will be more positive and healthy.

Food, Body Image, and Soul Satisfaction

Food in a very primal sense is about love. The very first way you attach to your mother (or primary caregiver) is through being fed as a baby. I've talked in previous chapters about how this initial relationship can be disrupted and can lead to insecure attachments. But you can also think about your attachment to food as a very real way in which you connected from birth onward to your parents and other familiar people in your life, and as a way in which you felt love. Think, too, of how many other purposes food has served in your life, as discussed in previous chapters. It's no wonder that when trouble arises in your life or when you want to celebrate something, you turn to food. It's mother's milk for your soul.

I've mentioned previously that food can often represent something that is missing in your life, and body dissatisfaction (or the desire to be thin) can do the same. When the deeper urges of your soul are not being met, it can feel as if you have a huge hole in your soul. You may have unconsciously tried to fill that void with food or distract yourself from the void by focusing on your weight. In the exercise below, see if you can identify the soul purpose you are using food and your desire to lose weight to fulfill.

EXERCISE: Metaphors for Soul Satisfaction

Answer the following questions to go deeper into your understanding of how food, body image, and weight issues have served as a substitute for soul satisfaction. List foods you tend to crave or binge on or foods you are afraid to eat for fear of gaining weight or for fear of not being able to stop eating once you start.

(Example: *When I eat strawberry shortcake, I feel comfort. It reminds me of my grandmother, and she was the person who I thought cared for me the most growing up. I usually crave this food when I am feeling stressed or lonely.*)

1. When I eat _____, I feel _____.

   It reminds me of _____.

   I usually crave this food when I feel _____

   or when I'm in a situation that makes me feel _____

   _____.

2. When I eat _____, I feel _____.

   It reminds me of _____.

   I usually crave this food when I feel _____

   or when I'm in a situation that makes me feel _____

   _____.

3. When I eat _____, I feel _____.

   It reminds me of _____.

   I usually crave this food when I feel _____

   or when I'm in a situation that makes me feel _____

   _____.

Continue deepening your understanding of your soul need associated with each food. If you were to look at how you feel and what situations or emotions lead to your eating or restricting the foods listed above, what might your true self really be looking for? What is your soul's need that you are trying to satisfy with each food? (*Example: My soul need for strawberry shortcake is a need for love or companionship, a need to feel like someone really cares about me.*)

1. My soul need for _____

   is a need for _____.

2. My soul need for _____

   is a need for _____.

3. My soul need for _____

   is a need for _____.

Now, let's look at what soul need you may have associated with body dissatisfaction thoughts. These thoughts may be about wanting to be thin, needing to go on a diet, or future projections of what being in a different body would mean to you.

1. Situations that trigger my longing to be in a different body include: (*Example: When I spend time with my friends who are married, I think about how my life could be different.*)

   _____

   _____

2. My future fantasy body would be: _____

   _____

3. If I had my future fantasy body, my life would be different in the following ways: (*Example: If I had a different body size, I would have a husband and a family.*)

   _____

   _____

   _____

4. When I think about my soul's need that underlies my desire for my future fantasy body, it is

☐ the need to be accepted

☐ the need to be loved

☐ the need to be noticed

☐ the need to be valued

☐ the need to be adored

☐ the need for safety

☐ the need for more joy in my life

☐ the need to feel I can express my sexuality

☐ the need for companionship because I am lonely

☐ to numb myself or self-soothe

☐ other: _____

5. What are the similarities and differences between how you use food to meet a soul need and how your body dissatisfaction is a way to meet a soul need?

Similarities: (Example: For both, I am looking for more love in my life.)

_____

_____

_____

Differences: (Example: I use food more for comfort when I'm stressed. My body dissatisfaction is more about wanting companionship or love.)

_____

_____

_____

The Road to Soul Satisfaction

If you've struggled with food and weight issues for most of your life, your self-worth may be inextricably tied to your weight (the number on the scale) or whether you've had a good-food or bad-food day—whether you ate what you thought you *should* eat and didn't eat foods you consider "bad" or fattening. Just like people whose whole focus is on making money, neglecting other important aspects of their lives, you may have decided at some point that the only way to have your needs for affection, attention, recognition, or success met is to lose weight. Think about how much of your time, energy, and focus (and money) has been spent on the pursuit of weight loss, perhaps sometimes at the expense of your relationships or other important goals. Just as the guy in pursuit of wealth will learn that making money doesn't determine his self-worth, you may also realize now that self-worth can't come from appearance, weight, or body shape or size. If it does, it will always be superficial and will not bring true happiness. True self-worth comes from your essence or your true self. You can tell the difference between true self-worth and superficial self-worth by paying attention to your feelings. When your life is a reflection of what you value most, what you love, you are more likely to be living a life of soul satisfaction. You can start by identifying what you truly value and then by recognizing how important it is to care for what you value most in the exercise below.

EXERCISE: Tending What You Value

For a moment, think about all the things that you value in your life. Perhaps you value family or your spouse, or perhaps you have a deep connection with your dog or cat. Maybe you value your work or your community involvement. Perhaps what is most important to you is your church community. Answer the following questions about your values.

1. My five most important values are: (*Example: I value my children, my work with the less fortunate at my church, my husband, having a welcoming home, and my dog, Sparky.*)

    • _____

    _____

- _____

_____

- _____

_____

- _____

_____

- _____

_____

2. How do you feel when you are doing or being with what you value most?

☐ I feel joy.

☐ I feel alive.

☐ I feel as if time flies because I am so focused on what I'm involved in.

☐ I feel safe and secure.

☐ I feel loved.

☐ Other: _____

☐ Other: _____

3. Next ask yourself if you are tending (caring for, cultivating) what you value most. List below the areas where you feel you are and are not tending what you value.

a. Areas of my life where I am tending what I value most include: *(Example: I feel I'm doing a good job with my kids.)*

_____

_____

b. Areas of my life where I am not currently tending what I value most include: (*Example: I realize that even though I value my relationship with my husband, I have put it on the back burner.*)

_____

_____

4. Now, regarding those areas where you are tending what you value, describe the ways you do that. (*Example: I spend time with my family and make our time together a priority even when there is pressure at work to stay late. I am committed to my work with the less fortunate through my church. I feed my dog a special food that I know is good for him, and I take him on frequent walks to help him stay healthy. I give my dog lots of affection.*)

_____

_____

_____

_____

5. For the areas you would like to nurture more, list below three small steps you can take to start tending these areas more thoroughly: (*Example: I want to start having date nights with my husband once a week to show him how much I care.*)

a. _____

b. _____

c. _____

Now that you know more about what you value in your life, you can use this information to help move you toward a life of soul satisfaction.

Accessing the Deeper Urges of Your Soul

When you shift your focus from the number on the scale to fulfilling your soul's needs, it shapes everything you do in life. For example, if your focus in your career is only on making money, you may pick jobs or a career that you don't love, just for the money. If you change your focus to finding work that satisfies your soul, you would look to do what you love for work. I've heard interviews with musicians, for example, who have said that they have not been able to stop making music even when they didn't make money because it was something they just loved to do. They chose the happiness and soul satisfaction that comes with doing what they love. In so doing, they also chose to live from their true self. Perhaps you have forgotten or left behind parts of your true self. Now is the time to reclaim that true essence and to begin the process of reclaiming the parts of yourself that have been ignored, forgotten, or left behind. Erica, for example, had put aside her desire to be a nurse. For you, it may be that you never felt you could handle having children—either out of fear that they might be hurt as you were as a child or because you felt that you would not be able to find the right partner unless you had the perfect body. Whatever parts of the deeper urges of your soul you put aside, now is the time to revisit those urges and listen to your soul's needs. In the exercise below, you will start the process that will help you do just that.

EXERCISE: **Who Are You Truly?**

1. Make a list of qualities you feel are part of your true self. Try looking at old pictures of yourself as a child for qualities that you may have forgotten. (*Example: I was always curious as a kid.*) You can also think of qualities that were important to you when you were younger or think of subjects or hobbies that interested you. (*Example: I always thought of myself as very athletic until I was nine and told by my coach that I didn't have the "right body type" to play soccer.*)

   _____

   _____

   _____

   _____

2. Take a moment to recollect the dreams you had when you were younger and thought anything was possible. Remembering that your soul-self can accomplish anything that it truly desires, what are those deeper urges of your soul, the dreams you had when you knew anything was possible that you want to bring

back into your life? (*Example: I want to learn to play the piano again. It was something I really enjoyed as a child but I haven't given myself permission to do since. I want to travel. I haven't allowed myself to travel because of my size, but I don't want to let that stop me.*)

_____

_____

_____

_____

3. List below the ways in which you may have deviated from your values, interests, and goals because of your focus on your weight or other issues in your life. List things you've put aside, waiting to lose weight. (*Example: I've been so focused on losing weight that I forgot how much I wanted to become a singer.*)

_____

_____

4. Now, make a commitment to yourself. By finding your anchor and accessing your inner strength, what can you commit to that would come from your true self? You may want to take some time to meditate on this and see if some truths bubble to your conscious awareness. You will know they come from your true self because they feel like a "lightbulb moment" or you may get a shiver of recognition when you think about them.

_____

_____

_____

_____

You can congratulate yourself for beginning the journey to soul satisfaction. Your hard work will pay off. You shouldn't expect to have mastered it all yet. This is a journey that will unfold over time with your ongoing commitment to healing.

PART II

Healing Yourself: Your Journey to Soul Satisfaction

In part 1, you worked through the levels of stopping surface behaviors, emerging from the emotional soup, embracing the wisdom of your body, creating new guiding principles, and finding soul satisfaction. Much of this work may have been emotional, but a necessary part of the healing process is removing blocks from the past and shifting the place from which you approach your desire to change your relationship with food and with your body—from that of the wounded self to your authentic or true self. If your desire to reach a healthy weight comes from the belief that being a certain weight is the only way to be happy, your efforts are destined to fail—as you may have noticed. When your desire is from a deeper, more authentic part of yourself, you will notice that your behaviors, thoughts, emotions, and core beliefs align. This alignment will enable you to be more aware of your choices, make choices based on your body's wisdom, and trust those choices, instead of doing what other people, even if they are considered experts, tell you to do. Most importantly, this shift will enable you to make more permanent lifestyle changes as opposed to following flash-in-the-pan diets that yield only temporary results.

In part 2, you will learn how to practice this new way of life—living from soul satisfaction rather than focusing on the number on the scale. Wouldn't it be great if you no longer felt upset when you looked at the number on the scale or looked in the mirror but instead could feel empowered, knowing that you are on your own personal path—one designed just with you in mind, one that uniquely fits your needs without ignoring your dreams? Wouldn't it be fantastic to be able to enjoy food again without fear or worry that you're eating the "wrong thing" or that you'll have to pay in some way for eating what you like? What would change in your life if you felt comfortable in your body and confident about your appearance because you knew on the deepest level that you are a worthwhile human being who deserves all that life has to offer? In part 2, you will find your path to true body satisfaction and food enjoyment and still be able to reach your healthiest weight—whatever that is for you. This transformation begins with a focus on nutrition and your relationship with food.

CHAPTER 6

Learning the Joy of Eating Well

Patti grew up in a home where she just didn't feel like she fit in. She was very bright and good in school even though no one else in her family valued education. She was also very sensitive emotionally, whereas her other family members didn't seem to have any emotions at all. She felt like an outsider. By middle school, Patti was overweight and her father began criticizing her about her weight. This was the beginning of her pattern of dieting to lose weight only to regain the weight she had lost and more. By the time she was in her thirties, she was obese. At age thirty-five, Patti decided to have gastric bypass surgery and lost over one hundred pounds. However, within three years, she had regained most of the weight she'd lost. When she started the Anchor Program, she weighed over two hundred pounds and was dissatisfied with her body and her inability to lose weight and keep it off. Her biggest hurdle was her diet thinking (thinking she had to skip meals and eat almost nothing to lose weight) and her aversion to eating vegetables. Patti also craved sweets and ate candy and baked goods on a daily basis. She started the Anchor Program and, as part of her evaluation, was tested for food sensitivities. She was found to have gluten sensitivity. She had a difficult time eliminating gluten foods, many of which formed her sweet treats. After one year in the Anchor Program, Patti had reached a weight she was comfortable with, and she was able to maintain this weight for more than two years. She felt good about herself and her body for the first time in as long as she could remember. During the program, she learned to eat three regular meals a day and one snack. Eating more protein helped curb her sugar cravings, as did understanding that sugar cravings were her response to stress. She learned new skills for coping with stress and reduced her reliance on food for stress management. She also finally decided to eliminate gluten from her diet. And amazingly, she couldn't believe that instead of craving chocolate, she was craving vegetables!

Nutrition is the foundation for improving the health of body, mind, and spirit. In this chapter, you will learn about the five components of the SIMPLE eating plan that takes the fear out of eating well, increases freedom around food, and reduces obsessive thinking about food. You will also learn about joyful eating. The joy of eating well is not just about what you eat. It's also about whether you enjoy what you eat, which is the more important thing. Joyful eating calls you to develop your palate and return to a mindful focus on food, silencing once and for all the critics and experts who tell you what to eat. The joy of eating well restores your individual tastes and body wisdom to its rightful role as the in-house expert that will guide you toward the weight that is right for you. So let's get started!

Joyful Eating

Joyful eating is about determining what works for you and your body, and learning to eat those foods with joy and without guilt or fear. The substance of joyful eating is not about what you eat. In other words, it's not about the food. It may be difficult at first for you to find a childlike curiosity about food and the willingness to put behind you the food rules of the past, and start fresh. Getting to joyful eating is a process that will take time, and at times you may feel like you've landed on a different planet entirely where the inhabitants don't focus all their energy on trying to change the way they look or the experience of eating, and where the conversations around food make people happy and carefree instead of anxious and sad. Perhaps you've had an experience similar to this when you've traveled abroad. I remember my first trip to Italy and how surprised I was to find that eating dinner could be a two-hour experience, with everyone eating freely, enjoying each other's company, and commenting on the taste of the different foods we were sharing. It was a real eye-opener for me. I've had similar experiences in many other countries I've visited.

Joyful eating is different for different people. It is not a diet in that there is no prescription to avoid or eat certain foods. There is no list of good foods or bad foods. This is because it is not what you eat, but how much and what is right for *your* body. Eating with joy entails finding an eating style that feels right for you. But more than anything, joyful eating is about listening to your body—not just listening to it tell you when you are hungry and when you're full. Your body has all the wisdom you need to determine what it needs to eat and when. Perhaps the more important aspect of joyful eating is allowing your body to use all of its senses to truly *savor the food* and *the experience of eating.*

You savor your food by paying attention to what you are eating and how it feels in your mouth and in your body. Do you like the taste of spicy food? Do you like certain flavors—savory, sweet, salty, rich food, bold flavors? To understand the experience of eating, you must pay attention to your environment. Do you enjoy eating with certain people? Do you like the ambience of certain restaurants, or do you want to set your own ambience at home—with candles and place mats, for example? Do you like trying new types of foods, ethnic cuisines, or unexpected flavors? Savoring the food and the experience of eating can be fun and exciting if you embrace the knowledge that you can trust your body's wisdom to guide you as you begin this shift to joyful eating.

Becoming a Joyful Eater

If you've been a chronic dieter most of your life and lived by food rules from numerous sources or if you are confused about what to eat, you may not be aware of how to listen to your body. You may not even regularly notice when you're hungry, for example. This may be because you skip meals, so your body has not become accustomed to any particular rhythm around eating, or you may have learned to shut out or ignore body cues of hunger. If you have the eating style where you snack all day long but don't eat regular meals, your body may not ever get the chance to send you a signal of hunger.

What follows is a structure that I have developed to help you learn to listen to your body. The SIMPLE plan is just that—a set of easy-to-remember guidelines to begin your journey to joyful eating. When you follow this plan, your body will begin to communicate (if you are ready to listen) to you about what to eat, when to eat, and when you are hungry or full. Once you become more proficient at listening to your body's communications, you can take it to the next level of joyful eating, which involves not just body cues of hunger or satiety but learning to eat for *satisfaction*. Your job is to follow the plan until you feel more comfortable making food choices, have more variety in your diet, and eat regularly throughout the day. After that, your next step is to start tasting the food you eat and noticing what you enjoy eating and what feels good in your body. This is the beginning of experiencing *satisfaction*, the most important aspect of joyful eating. Satisfaction is different from satiation or being full. You may feel that if you eat until you're full, that's all you need to do at a meal. But as you know, when you eat "rabbit food" or "diet food" or feel compelled to eat foods that you don't really want, you never feel satisfied. You may have a full belly, but your spirit is longing for something else—so you keep overeating. Finding satisfaction is the most important step you can take to become a joyful eater and involves truly enjoying the flavor, smell, and *experience* of eating. You may have incredible and surprising insights just as Patti did that you actually crave vegetables. You'll never know unless you leave behind your preconceived notions from the past and venture into the foreign land that is joyful eating.

Food Confusion Leads to Disordered Eating

As adults, most individuals with weight issues have been on numerous fad diets, read books on dieting and losing weight, and experienced the confusion of the expert recommendations that one minute promote low-fat diets and the next say don't eat carbohydrates or sugar. While there may be kernels of truth in expert nutritional advice, nutritional confusion also contributes to unhealthy eating styles. You may have dieting whiplash and just frankly have so much misinformation that you really don't know what is good for your body and what is not. So you end up eating lots of raw carrots and celery or stick mainly to salads. The advantage of what you are learning in this book is that you no longer have to pay attention to fads in the nutrition world; you have all the know-how you need to develop a healthy relationship with food by using your own body's wisdom and following the simple structure you are learning in this chapter. And instead of spending more money on fad diets, get a piggy bank and pay yourself some money for following your body's own wise food plan. Then, take a deep breath, throw out your diet books, and start to think about how it will feel to be free of all those confusing recommendations and of the fear and guilt you may experience around food now.

How Did You First Learn to Eat the Way You Do?

As a child, you heard either your parents or primary caregivers talk about food and eating or model for you certain eating behaviors. Ellyn Satter (2008, 1), a pioneer in analyzing eating behavior, states in her book *Secrets of Feeding a Healthy Family:* "Eating is more than throwing wood on a fire or pumping gas into a car. Feeding is more than picking out food and getting it into a child. Eating and feeding reflect our attitude and relationship with ourselves and with others as well as our histories. Eating is about regard for ourselves, our connection with our bodies, and our commitment to life itself. Feeding your child is about the love and connection between you and your child, about trusting or controlling, about providing or neglecting, about accepting or rejecting. Eating can be joyful, full of zest and vitality. Or it can be fearful, bounded by control and avoidance." This is a beautiful summation of the meaning food can have in our lives and exemplifies the message of this chapter—the importance of finding joy in eating well. It is also a reminder that not everyone has had the experience of joyful eating growing up.

Your adult eating behaviors, weight, and food preferences have their origins in childhood. If you grew up in a home where one of your parents tried to control what you ate, you are at higher risk for chronic dieting, binge eating, and eating disorders in adulthood (Birch and Fisher 1995). If your parents modeled healthy behaviors around food and provided you with a variety of foods, you are less likely to be overweight (Savage, Fisher, and Birch 2007). Every family has "family food rules"—some may be helpful, but many are harmful.

In the exercise below, you can start to identify all the rules you have around food from your family, the culture, and nutrition experts. Then you can decide what you keep and what you throw away.

EXERCISE: **Food Rules**

In this exercise you will identify the effect that your parents had on your eating. See if you can remember what your family food rules were and how your parents' modeling of these rules influenced your current weight and eating style.

1. Identify the family experiences that may have affected your current weight status and relationship with food. Answer the ones that apply to you. Add any other situations that were not listed that apply to you.

   • Growing up, my family didn't eat a lot of vegetables or fruits. This affected me by:

   _____

- My family used food as a reward with me ("If you're good, I'll give you a treat").

  This affected me by: _____

- My mother or father was always on a diet. This affected me by: _____

  _____

- My family never had regular mealtimes. This affected me by: _____

  _____

- I was put on a diet when I was very young. This affected me by: _____

  _____

- I always had to finish everything on my plate whether or not I was hungry.

  This affected me by: _____

- I was not allowed to eat sweets at home. This affected me by: _____

  _____

- Other family food rule: _____

  This affected me by: _____

- Other family food rule: _____

  This affected me by: _____

2. Identify all (and I mean all) the food rules you've learned from being a chronic dieter. Note things you've read in magazines or books and heard on the radio or television. You can include rules given to you by professionals—your doctor, your nutritionist, or your neighbor and best friend who think they are experts. I've included some of the more common ones to get you started.

   ☐ Skipping meals is the only way to lose weight.

   ☐ Eat six small meals a day.

☐ Low- or no-fat diets are the best way to lose weight.

☐ Avoid all carbohydrates in your diet.

☐ Fasting or doing cleanses is the best way to lose weight.

☐ Don't eat anything after 7:00 p.m. (or a certain time at night).

☐ Smoking keeps you from gaining weight.

☐ Pasta makes you fat.

☐ Dieting is the best way to lose weight (no matter what anyone tells me).

☐ Other: _____

☐ Other: _____

☐ Other: _____

☐ Other: _____

3. Look over the food rules you've learned from your family and from being a dieter. Ask yourself if any of them are beneficial for you. If so, keep those and work on eliminating the ones that don't help you. You can do this by being aware of when these rules come up in your life and countering them with a statement or affirmation that is more suitable for you now. An example of an affirmation you can use is "I don't need food rules; I have my body's wisdom." Write three food rules you'd like to eliminate and an affirmation that will remind you about your true self's goal to eat joyfully.

   a. Food rule I would like to eliminate: _____

       My affirmation: _____

   b. Food rule I would like to eliminate: _____

       My affirmation: _____

   c. Food rule I would like to eliminate: _____

       My affirmation: _____

Over time, you will find this enhanced awareness will create space for a new relationship with food to grow and develop. Now, you will learn more about a simple structure that gives you more freedom to enjoy the food you eat, without so many rules.

The SIMPLE Plan

While you may not be able to erase years of dieting knowledge, let's start fresh with a few simple habits. The SIMPLE plan is based on recommendations that have stood the test of time (and I don't mean six months!). These are recommendations that nutrition and medical experts don't debate because extensive research over the past fifty years has shown them to be true. I recommend that you explore each of the five steps below one at a time. The SIMPLE plan is designed to give you a starting structure so you don't have to *think about what to eat or think about food all the time.* This will create some space, time, and energy for you to learn to eat with joy. If you don't have to follow complicated instructions or count calories and fat grams, you will have opened up space to just taste what you are eating and also to create an experience of joy around eating. Remember, eating with joy leads to satisfaction, and feeling satisfied will alleviate the need to overeat.

The steps of the SIMPLE plan:

1. *Eat three meals and one snack daily.* Even the experts agree that eating every three to four hours is good for your health and good for your weight. When your body knows it can trust you to give it what it needs—regular nourishment—you will begin to feel hungry again. Eating regularly will also prevent spikes in blood sugar that lead to insulin release, which causes your body to store fat—especially belly fat. If you eat more frequently than three times a day or snack all through the day without eating meals, this recommendation will help you experience how your body feels when you allow it to feel hungry between meals.

2. *Eat protein at every meal and snack.* Eating protein regularly throughout the day is the secret to reducing cravings and controlling appetite. Protein helps your brain make the feel-good chemicals, such as serotonin and dopamine, that you need to stop cravings. You can choose animal or vegetarian sources of protein, which I will discuss in the seven-week plan.

3. *Eat at least three servings of vegetables and two servings of fruit a day.* Perhaps your mother turned you against vegetables by telling you not to leave the table until you "finish all your vegetables" or because she served up mushy versions of this important food group. For whatever reason, most of the people I work with who have weight issues don't like vegetables. Patti's story earlier in this chapter is an illustration of this and also of the fact that it doesn't have to be this way. Fruits and vegetables have many health benefits. If you think you "hate" fruits and vegetables, try them in different forms. I suggest you adopt a vegetable or fruit and see if you can eat it in its most natural state, as explained in the next step.

4. *Eat fresh and naked.* Learn to taste and enjoy food in its natural state—without added sauces, cheese, gravy, or other camouflage. That's not to say that you don't get to season your food. But try using fresh herbs, lemon juice, salt, and pepper. Eating fresh and naked allows you to really see which foods taste good to you and which don't.

5. *Stop counting calories.* Calories are simply units of energy. In our fat-phobic, diet-crazy world, just the word "calorie" has baggage associated with it. A simple way to determine how much you should eat without counting calories is the fist-and-palm method. One serving of protein should be the size and thickness of your palm. One serving of fruit, vegetables, or starch is approximately the size of your fist. Everyone's fist and palm are different sizes. So, using this method takes into account what your body needs. In order to determine the composition of your meal, refer to the plate method (http://www.nal.usda.gov/wicworks/Sharing_Center/NM/Plate.pdf), which advises that, to balance your meals, one-fourth of your plate has starch on it, one-fourth is protein, and one-half contains veggies, salad, or fruit.

With this structure in place, see if you can find your childlike curiosity to explore, savor, and experience different foods—even ones you may not have liked in the past. Be adventurous, and try to put aside your confusing rules about food from your past, which you will identify in the next section of this chapter.

Getting Started

In this chapter you've learned a lot about nutrition, without focusing on a particular diet. You've also learned to think more critically about food rules that came from your family or culture. You've also learned how important it is to search for satisfaction and find joy in eating. Eating with joy and satisfaction is an experience, not a to-do list. It's about being in the moment with your food—no matter what you are eating. It also involves suspending judgments you may have had about certain foods in the past, just as Patti did. Joyful eating is not about the past; it's about starting fresh and being present with the body you have today and what that body needs in order to be functional and happy. Joyful eating doesn't ignore the need for comfort or self-soothing, but it offers alternatives to solely using food for this purpose. Here are some steps you can use to immerse yourself in joyful and satisfied eating:

1. Provide structure to your eating plan by using the SIMPLE plan. This will supply a foundation that will give you time and space to begin normalizing your eating habits.

2. As you adopt the SIMPLE plan, begin to pay attention to your body's communications about hunger, fullness, the effect of the foods you are choosing, and your body's desires. Try to distinguish between what is an emotional want versus a body-wisdom-based need.

3. Stay aware of old rules about food from your family or culture, and decide which fit for you and which you want to discard. Try to stick with the SIMPLE plan and recognize when you are defaulting to old food rules or diet thinking (For example, *I have to skip meals to lose weight.*)

4. Taste your food, don't just eat it. Savor the flavors. See if you can identify spices and flavorings used in dishes you like. Try to categorize what you like about different foods.

5. Ask yourself before you eat, *What could I eat that would make my body happy?* Try the food you think will make you and your body feel good and see if you're right. If so, congratulate yourself. If you're mistaken, chalk it up to experience and keep experimenting.

In the next exercise, I recommend that you start to break down the components of this nutrition puzzle into bite-sized pieces. Start slowly. For now, focus on making small and permanent changes in your relationship with food.

EXERCISE: **Breaking It Down**

Make choices for steps you'd like to take and that you know are doable. Don't be overly ambitious. This is all part of a process. It's not a diet, where you have to change everything all at the same time. This is about going slowly and developing behaviors that will last a lifetime.

1. Start with one point of the SIMPLE plan to practice.

    *   Eat three meals plus one snack every day. (3+1)

    *   Eat protein at every meal and snack. (Pro@everyM/S)

    *   Eat three vegetable and two fruit servings daily. (3 veg, 2 fruit)

    *   Eat fresh and naked.

    *   Stop counting calories: use the plate method and the fist-and-palm method.

    After you feel you are consistently able to do one point, move on to another until you're consistently able to follow all five points. As you practice each step in the plan, remember to stay aware of the effect on your body of each change you make. Make notes on which foods your *body* likes (not your emotions or your mind, which thinks it knows what you should eat). You can do this in the journaling exercise below. You will know that your body likes what you are eating because you will feel energetic, not sluggish. You will also not have food cravings. If you find yourself craving sweets or other foods, it is likely that you are eating foods your body doesn't like or not eating enough of foods your body needs. For example, sugar cravings are usually a sign of not eating enough good protein. Your body will also show you what it likes by being hungry at appropriate times. For example, if you are hungry an hour after breakfast, you either didn't eat enough or didn't eat enough of what your body needs. It's an adventure. Just keep experimenting to find the balance your body needs. Along the way, listen carefully to your body's wisdom to learn what is needed. At the end of this chapter (and online at http://www.newharbinger.com/32127), you will find a food journal in which you can write your daily food intake and track your progress with the SIMPLE plan, along with the number of hours you sleep and how much exercise you get each day. Use this food journal in whatever way you choose. It is just a guide and shouldn't be something you feel you have to do. If you have a better idea of how to track your progress with the plan, use that instead.

Select *one behavior* you can change to make the experience of eating more joyful. Pick something you would *love* to do—not something that you feel you have to do or that is a burden. This is meant to be joyful, not dutiful! Approach this with an air of self-discovery. Ask yourself, *What would make me happy?* Here are some ideas to get you started:

☐ Eat at least one meal a day at the dining room table (instead of on a TV tray or standing up in the kitchen).

☐ Set the ambience for dinner by using candles or playing music.

☐ Eat with your eyes: set up your plate in an appealing and eye-catching manner.

☐ Take three deep breaths before you start eating, to clear your mind of the day's worries.

☐ Put flowers on the table.

☐ Pay attention to the taste of each bite of food as you eat it.

☐ Try different types of food you may not have eaten before to improve your palate. (How do you know you won't like it until you try it?)

☐ Practice being the last person at the table to finish your meal (eat more slowly).

☐ Other: _____

2. Keep an ongoing list of food experiences you've really enjoyed and what it was about the experience that was joyful. It may have been a meal in which you tried a new food and found it fantastic. It may have been the company you were with or the beauty of the food presentation. This is a way for you to learn what it means to eat with joy. It is also a call to mindfulness—in other words, being mindful of not just what you are eating but how you *feel* about what you are eating. Make this your diary of joyful eating.

I had the following joyful eating experience: _____

_____

_____

What made this joyful for me was: _____

_____

_____

I had the following joyful eating experience: _____

_____

_____

What made this joyful for me was: _____

_____

_____

I had the following joyful eating experience: _____

_____

_____

What made this joyful for me was: _____

_____

_____

Continue this practice (perhaps with the form available for download at http://www
.newharbinger.com/32127). I would advise you to keep a journal of joyful eating experiences over the next few months to years. I can still remember my most joyful eating experiences as far back as a decade ago. There was the tapas meal I had in Barcelona. Then there
was an incredible meal I had in Italy with my son—fresh-made pasta alfredo with garlic

bread, eaten on one of the many piazzas in Rome on a beautiful sunny day. And the list goes on. Make your own list and learn what makes you tick when it comes to the joy of eating well.

As you know, trying to do everything at once only leads to frustration. Not doing anything at all only leads to despair. The Anchor Program and specifically this approach to joyful eating have helped many people just like you change their relationship with food and with their body. If they can do it, you can too! To give you more direction, use the following week-by-week guide for the SIMPLE plan, which will also help you take the next steps needed on your journey to joyful eating.

FOOD JOURNAL

	MONDAY	TUESDAY	WEDNESDAY	THURSDAY	FRIDAY	SATURDAY	SUNDAY
Breakfast							
Lunch							
Dinner							
Snack							
Exercise							
# hrs Sleep							
daily ☑ list	3+1 ☐ protein @every M/S ☐ 3 veg ☐ fist+palm plate method ☐ 2 fruit ☐	3+1 ☐ protein @every M/S ☐ 3 veg ☐ fist+palm plate method ☐ 2 fruit ☐	3+1 ☐ protein @every M/S ☐ 3 veg ☐ fist+palm plate method ☐ 2 fruit ☐	3+1 ☐ protein @every M/S ☐ 3 veg ☐ fist+palm plate method ☐ 2 fruit ☐	3+1 ☐ protein @every M/S ☐ 3 veg ☐ fist+palm plate method ☐ 2 fruit ☐	3+1 ☐ protein @every M/S ☐ 3 veg ☐ fist+palm plate method ☐ 2 fruit ☐	3+1 ☐ protein @every M/S ☐ 3 veg ☐ fist+palm plate method ☐ 2 fruit ☐

103

CHAPTER 7

Learning to Move Your Body

Carol is a bubbly thirty-year-old woman from a large Italian family. Both of her parents are very overweight and have been on and off diets all of their lives. A typical conversation in their family is about the latest diet one or both of them wants to try and how Carol should join them on this exciting new quest for weight loss.

As a child, Carol loved to play soccer. She also rode her bicycle everywhere and enjoyed most athletic activities. At age eleven, at the end of the soccer season, her coach took her aside and let her know she wouldn't be able to be on the team anymore because of her weight. She was crushed and surprised because she was sure she was as good a soccer player as all of her teammates.

When she joined the Anchor Program at the age of thirty, Carol did well in all aspects of the program but seemed stubbornly opposed to exercising. It was during one of the group sessions when this resistance shifted. When asked about negative experiences around exercise, she remembered the experience she'd had at age eleven. She was able to identify with her younger self's sadness and the pain of losing her view of herself as an athlete. After that conversation with her coach, she had begun to believe that she could not be athletic because of her size and stopped being active at all. After working through some of the feelings from this traumatic experience, she realized that she no longer had to live by that belief and began to explore ways she could be the athlete she knew herself to be. She decided to ride her bike to work instead of driving. She also decided to try out for a softball team at work and really enjoyed playing competitive sports again. Carol was able to reconnect with her love of movement by identifying blocking beliefs that kept her stuck.

In this chapter, we move on to discussing a different aspect of your relationship with your body—specifically body movement. I use "body movement" instead of "exercise" because I know that the "e word" has lots of negative connotations. It has been co-opted by the diet industry just as food has—in other words, used only in the service of trying to get you to lose weight. No wonder just thinking about exercise may send you into a fit of resistance or may make you feel guilty that you're not doing enough or not doing the right kind—at least according to all the experts.

Just as I encouraged you to question the conventional wisdom that says you have to be thin to be healthy, or that some foods are "bad foods" and you should only eat "good foods," I am encouraging you now to turn your inner skeptic loose on the field of exercise and all its attendant "expert" advice. To begin, I will discuss the problems with exercise prescriptions that often keep heavier individuals standing on the sidelines. Then you will learn how to remove your personal exercise blocks and find enjoyment in moving your body again. This chapter will help you embrace your intuitive connection with your body's natural need to be in motion. This chapter is about allowing you to stretch and move your way beyond the yoke of exercise as a mandate for weight loss and into a new relationship with movement as the body's birthright.

To start our skeptic's journey to body movement, I'd like you to take a little trip down memory lane in the exercise below.

EXERCISE: **How I Learned to Crawl and Walk**

You may want to pull out an old photo album and choose three or more pictures of yourself at different ages, from toddler to age five, for example. Start by sitting in a comfortable chair with your feet flat on the floor. Take three deep breaths, breathing in through your nose and out through your mouth. Now bring your attention to the sensation of your breath *moving* through your entire body, from the top of your scalp to the soles of your feet. Imagine that your breath is moving through your body in the same way your body moves through life. You can imagine your breath dancing, swirling, stomping, and gliding through all the cells and organs in your body and as part of what connects your body to the vital energy that is life itself. Bring your attention now to the sensations in your feet. Now start to remember yourself as a child, thinking of the pictures you've found. If you have any issues with remembering yourself as a child, you can think of another child to use as a surrogate for this exercise. This may be your own child, a niece or nephew, or the child of a friend. As you go through the exercise, keep breathing and keep your attention on your feet.

1. Looking at each picture or thinking of a mental picture of yourself or of another beloved child, write down any memories you have of moving your body when you were a kid. Maybe one of your pictures shows you in motion, or you may have a mental image of yourself in movement. Maybe there's a family story you recall about your being active or liking certain activities when you were younger. If you are using a surrogate child, think of all the ways in which this child moves his or her body. The idea here is to capture the essence of how children (and you specifically) are in movement. Paint a picture that comes to life for you. (*Example: When I was a little boy, I used to wear capes and pretend I was a superhero. My mother has lots of pictures of me with towel capes, jumping off of benches and pretending to fly or running in the wind with the cape billowing out behind me. Later, there are lots of pictures of me climbing things. I didn't like traditional sports, but I loved doing cartwheels on the front lawn, swinging in the tire swing in our yard, and playing hide-and-seek in the bamboo forest in my backyard.*)

    _____

    _____

    _____

    _____

2. See if you can imagine the feeling of being in movement when you were a child, and describe that feeling. (*Example: I felt so free when I was running through the grass in my bare feet or when I would go swimming with my father and he would throw me off his shoulders into the pool. I remember laughing so hard I was hiccoughing when I would ride my bike down a hill, going as fast as I could on a dare from my brother. I felt excited and carefree!*)

    _____

    _____

    _____

    _____

3. Now ask yourself what made moving your body feel the way you described above. (*Example: I felt free because it felt so natural to be doing what I was doing. No one had to tell me I was doing it right or wrong. I was happy because I was doing what I wanted and loved to do.*)

_____

_____

_____

_____

Rediscovering the Natural Joy of Movement

You may be lucky enough to enjoy exercise—even if you are in a bigger body. You may have continued to play a sport you enjoy, or you may have the discipline of a marine drill sergeant and just make yourself do what you think you need to do. To you, I say: "Keep up the good work!" Maybe reading this chapter will help you encourage or be less impatient with friends or family members who don't feel the same way you do about exercise. But if you have food and body image issues, you may struggle with exercise. To you, I say: "Don't throw the baby out with the bath water." What I mean by that is don't let the voices of ex-coaches, parents, peers who teased you, or anyone else who robbed you of the joy of being in motion take away the pleasure inherent in moving your body. Don't let the voices of experts who told you that you will only lose weight by doing certain exercises stay in your head. Kick out of your mind anyone who told you, as Carol was told, that you couldn't do a sport or an activity you wanted to do because of your size! Let's bring the play back into movement and get rid of the idea that exercise is something you have to do. As a child, I remember spending all day every day "exercising" in the community pool in my neighborhood—but really all I was doing was playing with my friends. I remember riding my bike up and down hills trying to catch up with my brothers on their bikes. That could have been considered exercise, but to me it felt like just plain fun. Just as you can learn to eat with joy, you can also reclaim your right to move your body with joy. Moving your body is a natural desire that you have, or at least had when you were younger. For example, babies are in motion all the time, exploring their hands, trying to put their feet in their mouths, and trying to roll over—even when they don't know how. Toddlers start to stand up, eventually let go of coffee tables, and try to walk and then run as soon as they are able. Every time they fall down, they get up and do it again. Why? Because this desire to move the body is hardwired into our genes, and it takes a lot to make moving the body feel like something we *have* to do rather than something we *want* to do. In the exercise below, let's examine some of the ways in which your natural desire to move may have been corrupted to make you feel as though you need to "exercise."

EXERCISE: Exercise Messages

1. List below messages you got about exercise, body size, or weight. These could have come from family members, coaches, teachers, friends, or magazines and media sources. (*Examples: You can't lose weight by swimming. Or My physical education teacher told me I wasn't going to be a good basketball player. He meant I was too fat to be good.*)

   _____

   _____

   _____

2. Describe below all the "exercises" you have tried to lose weight and what the results were, along with how you felt about doing these exercises. (*Example: With every diet I go on, I try to do the StairMaster because I know it burns a lot of calories. I literally hate the StairMaster! Sometimes I'd lose weight, but most of the time, I'd get so frustrated with doing it that I would quit.*)

   a. Exercise: _____

   How I felt doing this exercise: _____

   How this worked for me: _____

   b. Exercise: _____

   How I felt doing this exercise: _____

   How this worked for me: _____

    c. Exercise: _____

    How I felt doing this exercise: _____

    How this worked for me: _____

3. Look at your answers to the questions above and see what insights and conclusions you can garner from your history of exercise. (*Example: I've never felt like I was very athletic. Because of this, I've always had to force myself to exercise and mainly only do it when I'm trying to lose weight. It's not a pleasant experience for me.*)

_____

_____

_____

_____

Good work! You may be thinking that no matter how hard exercising is for you, you still need to do it in order to be healthy and to reach a healthy weight. After all, exercise is good for you just like vegetables are good for you. Right? I would beg to disagree. You don't need to do exercise you hate in order to be healthy. Let's look at this a little more closely.

I Really Don't Need to Exercise?

I want to make the distinction again and again in this chapter between exercise and body movement. Exercise science is used to bury you in scientific information, such as how many calories an activity burns and how many minutes of each activity it takes to lose a certain amount of weight. Just as nutrition science has created a lot of food confusion, exercise science has turned our body's natural desire to be in motion into an experience that feels a lot like boot camp. And by the way, there are actually exercise regimens called boot camp, which promise to whip you into shape whether you like it or not.

Of course, moving your body is good for you. My contention, however, is that it doesn't need to be painful or make you unhappy! Just as depriving yourself of foods you enjoy leads to overeating or bingeing, forcing yourself to do exercises you think you should do rather than ones you love leads to high dropout rates and increasing resistance to moving your body at all. There's lots of good science that is meant to encourage us to move our bodies, but there's not much good science saying we have to do only certain activities. Brisk walking, ballroom dancing, leisurely biking, playing golf, gardening, and playing Frisbee are all examples of moderate-intensity activities that have positive health benefits (CDC 2014; Myers 2003; Pate et al. 1995; U.S. Public Health Service 1996).

When Joyful Body Movement Is Not Good for You

Body movement is not good for you when you don't do it. This is the most important take-home message from this chapter. If you don't move your body, you can't reap all the health benefits available to you no matter what size you are. Remember, it's not about doing something you don't like or forcing yourself to be active doing something you were told you "should" do. This whole chapter is about you rediscovering how natural it is to be in motion. When you read the examples of moderate-intensity exercise above, were you surprised that you could obtain health benefits and live longer by gardening or playing golf? Other examples include actively playing with your children, shoveling light snow, canoeing, and hand-washing a car. There are also jobs that include this type of health-promoting physical activity, such as waiting tables, working on a farm, picking fruits or vegetables, or delivering mail. Vigorous activities that you've been led to believe are the only ones that improve your health and well-being such as jogging, using a StairMaster, biking fast or uphill, and swimming laps are also available to you *if you want to do them*. But the bottom line is that the only "should" you need pay attention to is the importance of finding an activity you love and want to do, and sticking with it. Some physical activity is much better than none, and if you find a starting point doing something you love, you can build from there. For example, I took up tae kwon do and eventually traveled to Korea to study with my teacher's eighty-year-old teacher, ultimately getting a black belt. Trying something new brought me back to that feeling I had as a child that I was a physical being and that I loved moving my body. I just had to be open to choosing other ways besides the traditional exercises to do that. One of my clients began doing ballroom dancing and now competes all over the country. Another loves swimming laps in her mother's pool for an hour a day in the summer. Another has picked up weight lifting. Yet another client takes three to five yoga classes a week. Another does bike racing in the mountains and extreme bike rides (over fifty miles) with her husband. These are all people who are in bigger bodies who are doing something they love.

EXERCISE: **I Can't Exercise Because...**

If you've never been able to effectively initiate or sustain regular physical activity, it may be for some of the reasons listed below. See which you identify with and read the responses to each. Below each reason, write down any insights you have about how these apply to you.

1. *I feel embarrassed by my size and don't want to exercise in public.* This is a very valid concern experienced frequently by individuals in larger bodies. But there are always things you can do to make yourself more comfortable with your preferred form of exercise. If you would like to try yoga, for example, but are afraid you'll feel uncomfortable in a class setting, you could take an individual lesson. After one or two private lessons, you may find yourself less embarrassed. Or consider beginning with a simple walking program, building your confidence until you feel ready to join a gym. You can also ask a trusted friend to go with you to the gym or to a dance class so you won't feel so insecure.

   But I invite you to go beyond simple solutions to claim your right and privilege—no matter your size—to move your body, just as I advise you to participate more in life. I understand that being bold is not always easy, so you might need to work your way up to it. What I know from experience is that many of my overweight clients are hiding their enthusiasm for life, their creativity, and their natural gifts behind their weight. I encourage you to express yourself by allowing your body to move, dance, do a downward dog pose in yoga, or swim to your heart's content. Every time you step out and express yourself, it will become easier. It will also make it easier for the next heavy person to join your gym or participate in your yoga class.

   How does this apply to you? How can you relate? What are you moved to do about this issue so that you can move your body with joy?

_____

_____

_____

_____

_____

_____

_____

2. *I have health problems, and every time I exercise, I have pain, injuries, or other symptoms.* This can be a very real problem. If your motivation is strong but you are experiencing pain or other unpleasant symptoms after you exercise, I recommend that you work with a skilled personal trainer or physical therapist to ensure you are exercising safely. If you find that both motivation and physical limitations are at play, you may have developed a fear of hurting yourself, and that fear is sapping your motivation. The solution is the same. Working out with a qualified exercise therapist will help you get over this fear and start you on the road to success.

How does this apply to you? How can you relate? What are you moved to do about this issue so that you can move your body with joy?

_____

_____

_____

_____

_____

_____

_____

3. *I get bored exercising.* There are many people who find "exercise" boring. So don't exercise. Find other ways to move your body. If you define exercise as going to the gym and walking on a treadmill or biking for an hour, that may not be the best form of activity for you. Perhaps walking in the park or having swimming races in the pool with your children would be more fun. Remember, you're not looking for exercise as part of a diet program so you can lose weight in the short run. You're looking for a long-term, sustainable, enjoyable form of moving your body that doesn't bore you. I would suggest you keep trying different activities, look for something new and something that maybe you wouldn't normally consider, and see if it holds your interest longer. If you love doing something, you're more likely to do it on a regular basis.

    How does this apply to you? How can you relate? What are you moved to do about this issue so that you can move your body with joy?

    _____

    _____

    _____

    _____

    _____

    _____

4. *I don't have time.* In my experience, time is never the real issue. I'm sure you find time for anything you really want to do. Sometimes a lack of time as a reason not to exercise can signal the presence of an emotional block, which was the case with Carol in the story at the beginning of the chapter. We will discuss more about these emotional blocks later in this chapter. But just think of all the things you get done every single day. Ask yourself if all of them are top priority or if you can perhaps move some of them to the "if I get time" list and put physical activity higher up on your list. If you can find time to get your nails done, watch TV, and do other activities on your priority list, what would it take to make exercise a priority?

How does this apply to you? How can you relate? What are you moved to do about this issue so that you can move your body with joy?

_____

_____

_____

_____

_____

_____

Emotional Exercise Blocks

If you are still not feeling motivated to exercise your right to natural and joyful body movement, you may be like Carol in that you've had some exercise-related trauma, embarrassment, or past experience that has left you with an emotional block to moving your body. In Carol's case, she had not linked what happened with her soccer coach to her adult resistance to physical exercise. Becoming more aware of this enabled her to challenge the subconscious belief that she couldn't be athletic because of her size. It was a relief to her to be able to see herself as an athletic person again, and she quickly embraced physical activity for its own sake (because she loved to do it) rather than using it only in the service of losing weight. In the exercise below, you can explore the possibility of emotional blocks to moving your body.

EXERCISE: Challenging Emotional Blocks to Moving Your Body

1. List the feelings you have when you think of exercising or being physically active. (*Example: I feel angry.*)

_____

2. Make a list of experiences involving physical activity or exercise that led to the feeling(s) you mentioned above. See if you can understand what about the experiences led to the emotion. (*Example: I get angry when I try to walk on the treadmill because I remember the times I was told I had to do this to lose weight.*)

_____

_____

_____

_____

3. List below any other negative past experiences with exercise and the emotions you felt at the time. (*Example: I was made fun of in gym class. I felt ashamed and embarrassed.*)

_____

_____

_____

_____

4. List the beliefs and assumptions you made about exercising based on your answers to the questions above. (*Example: I was told I was too fat to be a dancer, and that's what I've believed. It kept me from taking dance classes or even dancing for fun because I felt so self-conscious about my body.*)

_____

_____

_____

_____

_____

5. Now, see if you can challenge those beliefs or assumptions by asking yourself if they are really true for you now. (*Example: There is no reason I can't be a dancer no matter what my size. I don't need to be a ballerina. I love jazz dancing; I love hip-hop. I love the thought of dancing to songs from the seventies.*)

_____

_____

_____

_____

_____

6. To help you release some of the pain from past experiences, go through the visualization below. (Repeat the visualization for each negative exercise experience.)

   Visualize yourself at the age when you had the negative exercise experience. Imagine your heart opening to allow your wounded self to receive your full love and compassion. Ask your wounded self what he or she needs to be made whole and complete and to release any emotions that may interfere with your body-movement program. Reassure your wounded self that you understand what he or she went through and that you appreciate the pain that was involved. Continue the process of offering kind and loving feelings to your wounded self. Ask whether he or she is ready to allow the old hurts to be put aside to allow you to experiment with body movement again. End the visualization when you are ready by giving your wounded self a sign of your appreciation, such as a hug or kiss or perhaps a smooth stone to keep in your pocket.

7. List three things you can do to reclaim your desire to move your body. If you are ready and willing, the act of actually doing some physical activity will help you heal emotional blocks to moving your body. Include a time for completion next to each goal. Also list any support you may need to help you complete it. (*Example: I will take one ballroom dancing class within the next three months. I'm going to ask my best friend if she'll take the class with me.*) If you feel you are not ready to explore body movement of any kind, list below any actions you can take to help you become ready. (*Example: I will continue to work on my trauma with my therapist until I feel more comfortable with the idea of moving my body.*)

a. _____

_____

b. _____

_____

c. _____

_____

Moving your body is a natural part of what it means to be human. When you feel resistance to something so natural, it may be because of trauma you've had in the past, some of which could be exercise-specific. You can use body movement to help you heal trauma. For example, there are trauma-specific yoga teachers who work with individuals who have post-traumatic stress disorder, a history of childhood trauma, or trauma related to natural disasters (Mitchell et al. 2014; Spinazzola et al. 2011; Staples, Hamilton, and Uddo 2013). You may find that moving your body, especially when it involves mindfulness (as in yoga, tai chi, and qigong) and breathwork, will enable you to be less uncomfortable in your body, to be more aware of your inner experiences and body sensations, and to better regulate your emotions and not be as triggered by traumatic memories (Van der Kolk 2006).

This chapter has hopefully helped bring to your awareness both how natural moving your body can be (says the child in you) and the ways in which past experiences may have blocked that natural joy in movement. Below are some tools for you to use when you are ready to take a leap into movement.

EXERCISE: **First Steps**

1. Select the steps you need to take to get yourself ready to start moving your body.

   ☐ Purchase appropriate body-movement clothing that is comfortable and attractive.

   ☐ Purchase appropriate shoes.

☐ Look at your calendar and schedule a time to do body movement on a regular basis. What days and times work best?

☐ Other: _____

_____

2. Decide how to begin.

☐ Take a class.

☐ Join a gym.

Names of gyms I want to check out: _____

What I am looking for in a gym membership (for example, an indoor pool or racquetball court):

_____

_____

_____

☐ Join a sports league (senior tennis or softball, for example).

☐ Set up one session with a personal trainer.

☐ Find a friend to work out with me. List potential workout partners:

_____

_____

_____

☐ Other: _____

_____

3. Choose some activities you would like to try.

- [ ] basketball
- [ ] walking
- [ ] gardening
- [ ] swimming
- [ ] yoga
- [ ] martial arts
- [ ] Pilates
- [ ] tai chi or qigong
- [ ] jogging or running
- [ ] skating
- [ ] other: _____

- [ ] dancing
- [ ] Nia
- [ ] Zumba
- [ ] tennis
- [ ] racquetball, squash, handball
- [ ] weight lifting
- [ ] ballet
- [ ] sailing
- [ ] playing with your kids
- [ ] cleaning your house

Great work! I hope you'll remember that moving your body is not something you have to do, so don't take the "marine drill sergeant" approach by forcing yourself to do something you don't want to do. Instead, see if you can tap into an inner feeling that draws you to a form of moving your body. It may not make sense to you, just as being interested in tae kwon do didn't make sense to me. But your body knows what it wants better than your intellect or mind. This is another way to tap into body wisdom. Follow your feeling, and stay open and curious. If you come up against embarrassment or body-image problems, look for a way around them. For example, if you are afraid of making a fool of yourself in a dance class, start by looking up dance videos on YouTube and then try a class. Remember, this is your body, and how you move it is your decision. But whatever you do, just move it!

CHAPTER 8

Learning Skills for Stress Management

Joseph is a forty-two-year-old man and the owner of a large business. He is married with two children in college and feels that his life is pretty good overall, with one exception—he is very overweight. He describes himself as having been "chubby" as a child. He participated in sports in high school and college, and he was able to keep his weight under control. However, after college, his weight slowly increased, and he now weighs over four hundred pounds. He has trouble flying because the seats are too small. While his wife doesn't complain about his weight, he feels she is less attracted to him. He has tried numerous weight loss programs, including inpatient programs, and he has no trouble losing weight. But he just can't keep the weight off. He realizes he is a stress eater. Running a large company leaves him little time to eat regular healthy meals or to exercise. The stress of his work and the financial strain of having two kids in college have taken their toll on him. Every time something goes wrong at work, he finds himself bingeing on junk food. His parents are aging, and he is the oldest in the family and the only one who lives near them, so he also is heavily involved with their care. This just adds to his stress and makes him feel hopeless that he will ever be able to get his weight down and keep it down.

In this chapter, you will learn about the important connection between stress and eating behaviors. If you are an emotional eater, stress can trigger emotions that you have been regulating with food. Joseph's case above illustrates how recurrent acute and chronic stress can sabotage any efforts you make to resolve your food and weight issues. Managing stress without food requires that you learn a new set of skills to use when you're feeling overwhelmed, worn out, or stressed to the max. Managing stress also requires learning to tap into your body's wisdom to identify the early warning signs and symptoms of stress, a key first step toward handling stress differently. Stress management involves a moment-by-moment mindful awareness that you may not naturally possess but that you can learn.

What Is Stress?

Stress can be difficult to define because it has so many causes and is different for different people. But you know what stress feels like, and you also have probably experienced how stress can wear you down—physically, emotionally, and spiritually. Sometimes stress is caused by a happy occasion, such as the birth of your first child and the subsequent sleepless nights that go along with that experience. If you are having a baby and it's not your first, your friends may tell you that you shouldn't feel stressed because you're an "old hand" at parenting. However, each of these experiences has its own reason for being stressful. In the first case, you may be inexperienced, nervous, and not sure about how to care for your first child. In the second, you may be caring for multiple children, which is a different kind of stress. Stress can be the result of pressure you put on yourself or pressure from an outside source. In Joseph's case, his expectations for success at work and the expectation that he must be the primary caregiver for his parents are major causes of stress. Another way work can be stressful is when you are afraid of failing, so you stress yourself out by overworking, trying to avoid that possibility. You may have a boss who is very demanding and is never satisfied with your work, or you may be in a job where you have little autonomy and very little input in your job—all of which are stressful. Stress is not all bad either. It can help motivate you to do your best work—up to a point. If you've ever competed in a sports event or had to meet a deadline at work, you know that this type of stress can be a strong motivator. Falling in love, buying a new home, and getting married are all examples of causes of stress (stressors) that are positive but nevertheless very stressful (Boudarene, Legros, and

Timsit-Berthier 2002; Coccia and Darling 2014). In all cases, when the demands put on you exceed your ability to cope, you will experience stress.

What is stressful to one person may not be stressful for another. Your perceptions and reactions to different situations are what make them stressful or not. Your perceptions are like wearing glasses with a certain color lens. If your lenses are red, then everything you see looks red. But someone else in your life may be wearing glasses with yellow lenses. When you say the chair is red, he says no, it's yellow. The glasses you wear have a certain color of lens because of your individual past experiences, just the same as the person who has yellow lenses has had different personal experiences. Increasing your awareness of the fact that each of us is wearing glasses with different-colored lenses will enable you to take your glasses off from time to time or at least to understand that your glasses aren't the same as someone else's and that the particular lens color is neither right or wrong. I'm mentioning other peoples' lens colors because so many of the life experiences we consider stressful involve other people—whether it be your spouse, your boss, your parents, or your children. The way they see things may be completely different from how you see things because of the color of their lenses. This applies also to whether another person sees certain situations as stressful. He or she is seeing the situation through his or her glasses, and you are seeing it through your glasses.

How Stress Affects Your Body and Leads to Disordered Eating

Stress is the number one cause of emotional overeating and bingeing. Some people consider stress the "pathway to obesity." If you have struggled with food and weight issues, you may be more likely to engage in overeating due to stress (Greeno and Wing 1994). If you have binge-eating disorder, you may be more likely to be an emotional overeater, and this may be one of the factors that can make you gain unwanted weight (Stice, Presnell, and Spangler 2002).

The stress response is mediated by the hypothalamic-pituitary-adrenal axis (HPA axis). The HPA axis is not the axis of evil, no matter how much you feel it makes you overeat or binge. It is how your body normally responds to a stressful event—either real or perceived as real—which makes you want to fight, flee, or freeze. Right after a stressful event, the stress hormones (cortisol, adrenaline, and noradrenaline) are released by a part of the brain called the hypothalamus. Initially, these stress hormones reduce appetite. This makes sense because if you are in a situation of perceived or actual threat, you can't stop to eat. Instead, your body uses stored energy (from the liver) to respond to the threat. If stress continues, the second set of stress hormones are released, preparing you to fight or run away. The end result is that blood flow is directed away from the gut to the muscles, and blood sugar, heart rate, and blood pressure increase. There are some negative effects of the stress response. For example, the stress hormone cortisol also suppresses the immune system, which may explain why you tend to get sick when under stress. Stress can also cause stomach upset, fatigue, muscle tension, headaches, urinary problems, changes in sex drive, and changes in sleep habits.

After the acute stress is dealt with, your body's production of cortisol will cause a spike in hunger and a desire to eat or binge. This too makes sense, because the energy you used to fight or flee has to be replaced after the stress is over. What makes this stress response problematic is when you are under chronic, long-term stress—either physical or psychological. In this case, your body continues to make cortisol, which continues to stimulate your appetite. Cortisol not only stimulates appetite, making you feel hungry all the time, it also makes you more likely to eat "comfort foods" and put on weight. Comfort foods are part of the body's inherent feedback system to help you return to balance. When stressed, you eat comfort foods that make you feel better for a time by stimulating the dopamine reward centers in the brain that were discussed in chapter 1. When you are stressed and you eat comfort foods, you are triggering the reward center in the brain, which releases brain chemicals that help you feel less stressed. So, eating comfort foods when you're stressed does work, but only temporarily. Repeated stimulation of the HPA axis through stress or eating comfort foods or both promotes the compulsive nature of overeating. So stress makes you want to eat, and eating helps your body regulate its stress response—a match made in heaven! This "perfect match" is then the cause of the food and weight issues that you are struggling with today.

EXERCISE: **I'm Stressed!**

The questions below are designed to help you identify your personal causes of stress and how you cope.

1. List below the things in your life that are causing you stress currently. I have listed a few examples to get you started. With each one, write specific reasons why you feel the situation is stressful for you.

a. Marriage (*Example: My husband is never around, so I'm always taking care of the kids plus the house by myself*).

_____

_____

b. Children _____

_____

c. Finances _____

_____

d. Parents _____

_____

e. Work _____

_____

f. Other: _____

_____

g. Other: _____

_____

h. Other: _____

_____

2. Now list physical, mental, or spiritual ways these stresses affect you. For example, you may get frequent colds or have back pain. Or you may be easily irritated or angry all the time. Or you may feel lonely and isolated.

a. Physical signs of stress: _____

_____

_____

_____

b. Emotional signs of stress: _____

_____

_____

_____

c. Spiritual signs of stress: _____

_____

_____

_____

3. How do you use food to deal with your stress? Describe what types of food you eat under stress, how much, and how you feel before and after. Think of other ways stress can affect your weight. How does stress affect your body image?

_____

_____

_____

_____

_____

_____

As you can see, stress has a lot to do with food and weight issues. The stress you are experiencing currently can affect multiple areas of your life. Another aspect of stress comes from the stress you may have experienced earlier in life, which you'll learn about next.

How Early Life Stress Contributes to Food and Weight Issues

Not only can chronic stress in adulthood worsen food and weight issues, early life stress can play a potent role as well. You've learned in previous chapters that toxic stress in childhood can have an effect on the hardwiring of the brain itself. Early life stresses actually change the genes that affect hormones that control eating behaviors, the feeling of fullness (satiety), and appetite. These hormones include ghrelin, leptin, and insulin. Early toxic stress causes changes in the brain that thereby change eating behaviors long-term, not just in childhood. These changes can cause cortisol levels to be consistently high—even when you're not under stress (Adam and Epel 2007; Sominsky and Spencer 2014).

Personality traits and coping styles can also have a direct influence on how you perceive stress. For example, if you tend to be a very anxious person or someone who worries about everything or always expects things to go wrong, you may be more likely to see situations as stressful than someone who is less anxious or depressed. But stress can also cause anxiety and depression, which then makes it harder for you to cope with ongoing stress. The interaction between mood and stress is therefore a vicious cycle. One leads to the other and vice versa. If you have suffered some kind of loss in your life, such as the death of a loved one, a separation or divorce, or even the threat of separation, you may develop depression within months of such an event (Paykel and Cooper 1992). Other types of losses that may cause you to become depressed or anxious include the loss of a role you've been playing in your life (wife, mother, executive), loss of self-esteem or status, or loss of your country or culture (as with refugees who are forced to leave their homeland, for example; Brown, Harris, and Hepworth 1995; Shalev et al. 1998).

What Determines How You Cope with Stress?

Social support is an important factor in how you cope with stress. Social support can mitigate the negative effects of stress in your life—whether you are a college student, a person diagnosed with cancer, or pregnant and at risk for a premature birth. As you may have experienced in programs such as Weight Watchers, social support can also help children and adults improve their weight loss efforts and reduce perceived stress (Cho et al. 2014; Goldschmidt et al. 2014; Yardley et al. 2014). Social support can come from your family members, friends, clergy, teachers, therapists, coaches, and many other sources. Tapping into sources of social support is important in managing stress and helping you cope with food and weight issues.

What Causes Stress?

Events or situations in your life that cause stress are called "stressors" and can include events such as loss, separation, and divorce. Other potentially stressful events you may have experienced include personal injury or illness, being fired at work, financial problems, illness in a family member, changing careers, marriage, retirement, pregnancy, buying a house, a child leaving home, getting a promotion, and many more. If you have any significant change in your life, it can potentially cause stress.

What is it about change that causes stress? If you think about it, change is only stressful if you resist or try to avoid the change. This would mean that you have a judgment about what is happening—it's good or bad, it's right or wrong, or it should be this way, not that way. You may think of this as the most natural thing in the world. "Of course, I think _____ is bad. Everyone I know does too." Buddhist philosophy states that while pain is part of the human condition (the Christian version of which is "everyone has their cross to bear"), suffering is not. One cause of suffering is ignorance, or not seeing the world as it actually is (rose-colored glasses), which we discussed above. Suffering is also caused by nonacceptance of pain or wanting things to be as they are not, which is sometimes called craving. We want our partner to be different, or we want to change ourselves. The causes of stress are the causes of suffering.

To describe it more fully, something *changes* (or threatens to change) and there is *stress*, then we *react* (have emotions and *judgments* and either accept the situation or not). If we choose to *surrender* to the reality of the situation, there may be pain, but not as much suffering. If we are in *nonacceptance* mode, there is suffering, and the stress attached to this situation worsens.

The pain that all humans experience is caused by situations that we have no control over or that we judge. I call this type of pain "the pain ball."

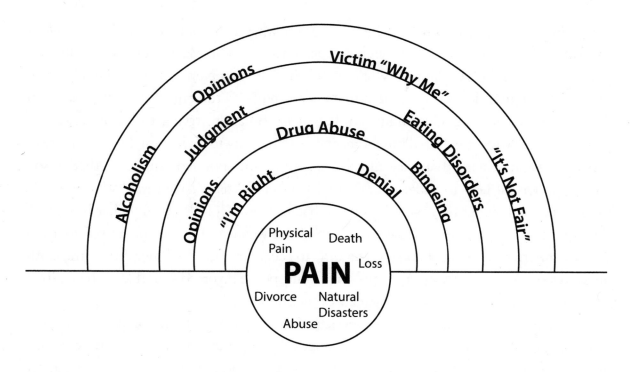

Think of the pain ball as a large expandable ball that each of us carries with us. You can imagine this ball sitting beneath your heart and right in the middle of your solar plexus (in your upper abdomen), considered to be the seat of your personal power. This metaphor is very apt if you think of how much of the pain you experience in life has to do with your heart breaking or feelings of helplessness (or powerlessness). Even positive stressors affect the heart and the power center. If you have a baby, your heart swells with pride and you feel powerless at times to protect your child from life's little and maybe big traumas.

In the pain ball is loss, divorce, physical illness, trauma, abuse, neglect, and any other painful experiences that you have gone through. The pain ball illustrates how suffering takes what is already painful and magnifies it through nonacceptance of the situation or wanting things to be as they are not. In the diagram, you can see some examples of things that can create pain in the pain ball, along with examples of ways in which our perceptions can lead to suffering. You may have different items in your pain ball or have different examples of what causes suffering in your life. The most important point is for you to become aware of the difference between pain and suffering. For example, if you have gone through a divorce, you can either spend your time working on the pain from this loss—letting go of your dreams for your marriage, dealing with sadness that accompanies such a loss, expressing your anger—or you can try to avoid all this pain (sometimes using food to do so) by spending most of your energy telling yourself, *It didn't have to happen; he shouldn't have done this or that; if only he could have done such and such.* Maybe you can see the difference between the two options. Working on what's in your pain ball—whether it's something from your childhood or something more current—is the only way to alleviate pain and minimize suffering. Continuing to judge your situation; trying to fix or change it; making others wrong; manipulating someone or something to make him, her, or it more of what you want; denying that something is happening; and trying to control another person or a situation all lead to suffering. Spiritual teacher Eckhart Tolle says: "Whatever the present moment contains, accept it as if you had chosen it" (Tolle 2015). What he's advising is that you work your way toward acceptance of whatever life presents to you to avoid further suffering. This is not about pretending to accept; it's about telling yourself the truth in each situation so that you can move on. If your spouse divorced you, that is the truth of the situation. Everything else is what causes the suffering.

Now, you are not alone if you experience this kind of suffering or if you feel that accepting certain situations is completely impossible. It's human nature to have complex reactions to various stressful circumstances. It's human nature to want someone to pay for your pain. However, if you can become aware of how suffering is more under your control than pain is, you have the ability over time to lessen your own suffering by recognizing that healing requires acceptance at the deepest level possible.

You learned about this deep level in chapter 5 when I talked about soul satisfaction and living more from your authentic self. The authentic soul self wants healing above all else—even above payback. Our smaller or nonauthentic self is happy to play the blame game, to be just plain stubborn, or to feel stuck in a victim role. When you commit to living from your authentic self, you are also committing to healing old and new wounds in a way that makes you the most whole. In the exercise below, you will be able to experience this in a more in-depth way.

EXERCISE: **The Pain Ball**

Checkmark experiences you've had or are currently having that should be included in your pain ball. These are experiences that you would consider part of what it means to be human. Try to leave out emotions, judgments, opinions (for example, anger or being mistreated), and anything else that has to do with perception. I've given you some ideas to get you started.

My pain ball includes

☐ death of a pet

☐ loss of a loved one (human)

☐ divorce

☐ physical illness or chronic physical pain

☐ physical or emotional abuse

☐ sexual abuse

☐ physical illness in a loved one

☐ disability in a loved one

☐ other: _____

☐ other: _____

☐ other: _____

Next, checkmark the ways that you may have created suffering in your life in an attempt to control the situation, avoid it, or deny it—in other words, ways you've tried to avoid dealing with the pain in your pain ball.

☐ I have held on to anger, sadness, or regret.

☐ I have been in denial about the problem, pretending it doesn't exist.

☐ I have used food to numb my emotions.

☐ I have used other substances (drugs, alcohol).

☐ I have used other behaviors to deal with my problems (gambling; bingeing; purging; use of laxatives, diuretics, or diet pills; sex; or sex addiction).

☐ I have been very judgmental about people or situations in my life.

☐ I have used my emotions to manipulate others.

☐ I have played the victim role (different from having been victimized) to manipulate others.

☐ I have made excuses for my negative actions.

☐ Other: _____

☐ Other: _____

☐ Other: _____

Describe, in as much detail as possible, one of the situations in your pain ball that still has some emotional charge attached to it. Then answer the following questions to see if you can gain a better understanding of how you have coped with the stress of what's in your pain ball. (*Example: My father died ten years ago, and I feel like it was just yesterday. I was just finishing physician assistant school and came home for spring break and found out he had been complaining of chest pain and indigestion for a few weeks. He had been given treatment for indigestion that hadn't helped, and he had also gone to the emergency room but was discharged and told he had an ulcer. By the second day I was home, he had a massive heart attack and died in the ambulance on the way to the hospital.*)

_____

_____

_____

_____

_____

_____

What are your judgments about this situation? (*Example: I am mad at the doctors who took care of him because they didn't seem to care whether he lived or died. I don't think the hospital emergency room should have discharged him when he went in the first time. My stepmother didn't take his complaints seriously enough. He should have gotten medical care sooner.*)

_____

_____

_____

_____

_____

_____

How have your judgments kept you stuck in suffering? *(Example: I've been sad about this situation for a long time. Then I get angry when I think about what should have been done to help my dad. I feel like he shouldn't have died. I feel caught in a vicious cycle.)*

_____

_____

_____

_____

_____

What emotions are you trying not to feel about this situation? *(Example: I don't want to feel the guilt. I am okay feeling sad or even angry, but deep inside, I feel guilty and also helpless. I think I should have been able to do something to save my dad. After all, I'm a physician assistant. I should have been able to help him.)*

_____

_____

_____

_____

_____

How has this situation affected your eating, weight, and body image? *(Example: When I think about my dad and all the emotions come up, next thing I know I've eaten a box of cookies or a carton of ice cream. I've put on a lot of weight since his death, and I can't stand the way I look.)*

_____

_____

_____

_____

Now take three deep breaths, grounding yourself by putting your attention on the inner sensations of your feet, which should be flat on the floor. Take another three deep belly breaths and feel the energy of your breath moving from the top of your head to the tips of your toes. Next, answer the questions below.

What does your authentic soul self *need* in order to resolve or let go of the suffering you're experiencing around this situation? *(Example: I just want him to know how much I love him. I didn't have a chance to tell him before he died. I've been haunted by not being able to see him again and tell him how much I love him.)*

_____

_____

_____

_____

What can you do in this moment to address your soul's need for healing? *(Example: I can write him a letter letting him know how much he meant to me, and I can then bury it under the big oak tree he planted when I was born.)*

_____

_____

_____

_____

Again, take three deep breaths, keeping your attention on the inner sensations of your feet, and write the *truth* about this situation. Your truth will come from your soul self. Your truth will not have anything to do with judgments. Rather, it will be a summary statement of the essential truth that will free you from the vicious cycle of suffering and allow you to move forward in your life. When you arrive at this essential truth, you may feel as if a burden has been lifted from you.

(*Example: I know my father knew how much I loved him. It's also true that even with all my medical knowledge, I can't save everyone. I also know my father wouldn't have expected me to punish myself for his death. He would want me to get on with my life and honor him by enjoying life again.*)

_____

_____

_____

_____

After completing this exercise, take three more deep breaths, releasing any remnants of emotion or tension in your body. Scan through your body mentally and allow yourself to fully relax, knowing that you have done the right thing. Letting go is a healing practice that reduces suffering and enables you to cope better with stressors in your life. Recognizing stressors, especially those that have been stuck for some time, is the first step toward a fresh start in which you recognize that you are worth healing, that you are much bigger than any of your problems or any toxic experiences from your past. When you allow your authentic soul self to direct you, it will always move you toward the whole, complete, beautiful being that you are.

Other Ways to Manage Stress

You've just learned about the deepest practice for stress management, which I'd like to reiterate for you here before we move on.

1. Identify your judgments about the stressor.

2. Don't stuff your emotions—just let them be, and feel them.

3. Ask yourself what the truth of the situation is.

4. Let go of all else but the truth.

5. Release tension from your body.

You may not need to use this process for smaller stressors, or you may use this process and find that the stressful feelings continue to come back; in other words, for more difficult situations, this won't relieve your stress right away. If that's the case, here are a few other techniques you can use to help manage your stress.

Adaptogens

Adaptogens are herbs and other supplements that help your body resist the damaging effects of stress. Following are a few of my favorites.

Panax ginseng has been used in Asia for centuries, and its benefits include improved physical stamina and endurance, blood sugar levels, and immune function (Shergis et al. 2013). You can also take *P. ginseng* to help with memory, concentration, thinking, and mood (Kennedy, Reay, and Scholey 2007; U.S. National Library of Medicine 2014).

- *Side effects*: usually minimal but can include trouble sleeping. *P. ginseng* should not be taken by children, pregnant women, or individuals with any autoimmune diseases. If you are taking prescription medications, you can check with your doctor before taking *P. ginseng*.

- *Dosage*: 200 mg per day. You can also use *P. ginseng* tea or tincture. The tincture does contain alcohol so should not be used by alcoholics.

Aromatherapy involves the use of essential oils and has been used to reduce stress by many people. If you are experiencing work-related stress, you may want to try using lavender oil that you can put on a handkerchief pinned to your uniform or use in a diffuser in your office (Chen, Fang, and Fang 2013).

Other Techniques

Breathwork includes many different forms of breathing consciously. You can count your breaths. You can breathe in to the count of four and exhale to the count of eight. You can focus your attention on your breathing. You can also inhale positive feelings and exhale negative feelings. Breathwork is also included in activities such as yoga, tai chi, and qigong.

Grounding techniques can help you gain a little distance from your stressor. Using your senses, look at objects around you one by one, noticing details of each. You can also feel the sensation of the chair beneath you and your feet on the floor and put your attention in your feet as we've discussed in previous chapters.

Self-care techniques help you deal with stress and prevent it from becoming overwhelming. These include all the alternative therapies such as acupuncture, massage, chiropractic, energy work (Reiki or Healing Touch), and so forth. If you know you will be entering a stressful period in your life or if you are in a very stressful period, you can schedule, for example, a massage once a week or every two weeks. If you're concerned about the cost, look for schools of massage or acupuncture, for example, where they offer discounted treatments.

Having a daily practice of self-care is also helpful. This could be taking a bubble bath at night to calm yourself, using aromatherapy, sitting or walking in nature, or going out with friends. It could also involve a daily prayer or meditation practice. Sometimes drawing or painting is a release from stress. Regular physical activity is also an option. More than anything, finding or making time to have some fun each day is a big stress reliever. This could be something as small as listening to the comedy channel on the radio or watching a happy, heartwarming movie.

Stress is unavoidable. How we manage stress is the only thing we can control. By recognizing when you are stuck in the vicious cycle of suffering caused by your perceptions and judgments of a situation, you can begin to reduce the stress in your life. Learning new techniques and daily practices will allow you to deal with stress without turning to food for comfort and relief.

CHAPTER 9

Learning to Nourish Your Spirit

Natalie is a very successful realtor but has struggled with her weight since the birth of her son, twelve years ago. She put on over sixty pounds during her pregnancy and afterward continued to gain. Her husband was diagnosed with a chronic illness when her son was just five and after that was no longer able to work in his construction business. Natalie was suddenly the only wage earner in her family, caretaker of her husband, and essentially a single parent. Now, she doesn't have any time for herself. Her work seems meaningless, and she can't seem to find a way to get back to feeling happy in her life. She runs from work to pick up her son from school and then home to help him with homework, take care of her husband, and fix dinner for the family. By the end of the day, she is exhausted. She hasn't had a vacation in over five years and can't even seem to find time to get a manicure or go to lunch with her girlfriends. In fact, she's lost track of most of her friends. Her weight has ballooned to over three hundred pounds. She knows she needs to take better care of herself, but she can't figure out how she will ever find the time. Life seems like a vicious cycle with little joy or happiness.

In the last chapter, you learned how stress affects your body, mind, and spirit and how stress can contribute to emotional overeating. You also learned about the pain ball and the importance of acceptance of what is, rather than judgment, in order to reduce suffering in your life. One of the ways to become more resilient and less reactive to stress is to nourish your spirit. If you think of times when you were spiritually depleted, just as Natalie's story illustrates, you know how hard it was at that time to just get through each day, let alone cope with any extraordinary stressors in your life. Nourishing your spirit is good preventive medicine for stress resilience, but it is much more than just a way to help you cope with stress. Nourishing your spirit enables you to stay more present to whatever is happening in your life, which will help you make better decisions and help with emotional regulation. Nourishing your spirit is a way to replenish what the world takes out of you, a way to keep your "cup full," so you can not only give to others in your life, but most importantly, give to yourself.

The chaos of modern life makes it difficult to know how to connect to your spirit. You may have been using food to try to "feed your soul." But the nourishment needed by your spirit is not food—it is self-love. You can't nourish your soul by focusing on things outside of yourself—the perfect body or relationship or job or even taking care of everyone else at the expense of yourself, as Natalie did. To nourish your spirit, you have to turn inward to the deeper meaning that life offers rather than look to the superficial values society worships or to the expectations that you have put on yourself or that others have put on you.

In previous chapters, you've learned about some of the ways in which trauma, abuse, and neglect may have impacted your physical and mental health. There is also a deep connection between spiritual well-being and health.

Spirituality and Well-Being

Native American cultures believe that illness is caused by spiritual problems, and Native American healers use herbs and rituals to restore a person to a healthy and spiritually pure state. Western religions also address the effects of spiritual depletion. For example, the Bible (Prov. 18:14) states: "The human spirit can endure in sickness, but a crushed spirit who can bear?"

Although your medical doctor may not have discussed the need to nourish your spirit for good health and well-being, some very specific benefits are associated with spiritual well-being. Just as toxic childhood experiences are associated with negative changes in your brain, spirituality and religion are associated with positive changes in your brain, which can reduce your risk for depression and also improve your recovery from depression (Miller et al. 2014; Peselow et al. 2014). This benefit can have direct effects on your eating habits and weight, given that people with depression may be more likely to binge eat or have problems with their weight. If you are Hispanic or African American and consider yourself religious or spiritual, you may find that you respond better to spiritually based weight loss interventions than those that are more secular (Davis et al. 2014; Nam 2013). If you experience a lot of body shame, you may be surprised to know that nourishing your spirit can not only help you reach a healthy weight but also reduce disordered eating behaviors and decrease body shame (Boisvert and Harrell 2013). If you are a yoga enthusiast, this spiritual discipline and the associated exercises can help improve eating attitudes and body awareness. Yoga also reduces body dissatisfaction (Dittman and Freedman 2009).

In previous chapters, you've learned about the importance of being present in your life and not going through life on autopilot. The rituals and behaviors associated with nourishing your spirit invoke mindfulness and can help you train your mind to be more flexible and adaptable, improve emotional regulation, and increase your ability to be attentive. If you are spiritually well nourished, you may not feel as stressed and may be able to cope better with any stress you do have (Tuck, Alleyne, and Thinganjana 2006). Finding meaning in something greater than yourself promotes happiness, and if you are happier, you're more likely to be healthier (Paulson et al. 2013). Nourishing your spirit should, therefore, improve your overall physical and mental well-being and bring joy and energy into your life.

Spiritual Depletion

Being out of touch with or disconnected from your spirit can lead to spiritual depletion. Toxic relationships, betrayals of trust, and chronic illness in yourself or a loved one are other experiences that can cause your spirit to be depleted. Being spiritually run-down can sneak up on you, and you may not even recognize the signs. Spiritual emptiness is a sickness that has signs and symptoms just like any physical illness. It's important that you recognize the signs so you can address the causes of spiritual depletion with as much compassion and care as you would any other illness. Below are some of the common signs that your spirit is in dire need of nourishment.

The Hole

One sign of spiritual depletion is the feeling that there is a hole inside of you that makes you feel somehow incomplete or "not enough." You may be turning to things, behaviors, and people trying desperately to fill this hole. Or you may have turned to food, alcohol, drugs, sex, or relationships to fill that hole. For example, if you have been working very hard to overcome your food and weight issues, you may have found yourself drinking too much or gambling or using drugs. Perhaps, you eventually got your drinking somewhat under control, and you then started acting out sexually—being promiscuous or even more demanding sexually in your marriage. Sometimes this can go to extremes, and you may cheat on your spouse or start looking at pornography on the computer. It's all an attempt to fill that hole. But the hole is a sign of a spiritual, not physical or emotional, emptiness. Spiritual emptiness can cause you to feel lost and alone. It can make you feel as if life has no meaning or purpose. You may find yourself thinking that life is not worth living if you can't be thin or find someone to love you or have more money, or if you can't…fill in the blank. But this hole is one that will not be filled by something outside yourself—no matter how many times you find what you think you want. Only you can fill this hole. Only you can do this for yourself. That's the good news and the bad news. It's good news because if you are willing to nourish your spirit, you will be able to live a fulfilling life, free from the void. It's bad news because there's no magic pill. No one can do it for you. Later in this chapter, you will learn more about how you can fill this hole.

Restlessness

Besides the hole, another sign of spiritual depletion may be restlessness to the point that you may feel the need to change jobs, leave your relationship, or move to a different city. You may feel like you're coming unglued or like you want to jump out of your skin. Your life may begin to look all wrong to you. Again, these are signs of spiritual depletion, and if you change the outside (your life circumstances) without changing the inside (by nourishing your spirit), you will find yourself back in the same situation in short order. If you're in this type of pattern, you may have tried the "geographical cure" by moving to escape a failed relationship or to get away from another bad situation. If you look back on those times now, you may realize that this type of change on the outside didn't fix the internal problem you were struggling with. It's only by digging deeper and recognizing that restlessness may not be a reason to leave; rather, it may be a call to action to make changes in yourself, not your situation.

Hopelessness

You have experienced one of the most common signs of spiritual depletion if you've felt hopeless. Hopelessness can be defined in many ways; it can manifest as a lack of hope, a sense of despair, or feelings of desperation. If you feel hopeless, you expect only negative things to happen in the future. You may also feel that you are helpless to make any changes in your life (Marsiglia et al. 2011). For example, if you've been on the diet treadmill most of your life, you may have felt hopeless that your weight and body image issues would ever change to your satisfaction. This is a train of thought that can lead you to depression and can negatively affect your self-esteem and sense of self-worth.

Hopelessness has repeatedly been shown to affect overall physical and mental health and well-being. If you experience high levels of hopelessness in your life, you are much more likely to develop high blood pressure or heart disease or to have a stroke, for example (Haatainen et al. 2004; Whipple et al. 2009). If you are male, especially if you are single, divorced, or widowed, you have a higher risk of hopelessness (Everson et al. 2000; Haeffel et al. 2008). Hopelessness can lead you to feel suicidal, or it can make you just feel trapped. If your situation has progressed to the point that you are having suicidal thoughts, you should call a suicide hotline in your area or talk with a therapist or medical doctor. Sometimes, external support is necessary to get you back on track. So don't feel bad if you need that support. Use what works for you to heal, and continue to look for ways to nourish your spirit.

Loss of Passion and Purpose

If you feel as if you've lost your passion and purpose in life, you may also be in dire need of spiritual nourishment. You may feel a deep longing for there to be more in your life, and you may feel like you're not living up to your potential or that you need to find a bigger purpose in life. Or you may find yourself asking existential questions such as, *Why am I here?* and *What is life all about?* All of these are symptoms of the need for spiritual nourishment. Well-known Austrian psychiatrist and Holocaust survivor Viktor Frankl wrote about his experience in the concentration camps in his book *Man's Search for Meaning* (1992). He defined the primary purpose of life as the search for meaning in whatever circumstance you find yourself. According to Frankl, if you have purposeful work, love, and courage in the face of life's difficulties, your life will have meaning. The value of love as described by Frankl is the very type of love that nourishes the spirit. It is a love of another's (and one's own) spiritual being or essence which transcends even death. You can find meaning in many aspects of your life and also in suffering. The way in which you address suffering in your life is what gives life its meaning, according to Frankl. Having courage in the face of difficulty is not always easy. If your life feels out of control or overwhelmingly stressful or if you feel backed into a corner with nowhere to go, Frankl's ideas urge you to remember that you still have the freedom to choose how you respond to the situation you find yourself in. As you choose how you respond, as you dig for courage to heal, and as you care about others and perform meaningful work, you will be nourishing your spirit.

In terms of finding meaning through your work, Steve Jobs, in his 2005 Stanford commencement speech, said: "Your work is going to fill a large part of your life, and the only way to be truly satisfied is to do what you believe is great work. And the only way to do great work is to love what you do. If you haven't found it yet, keep looking. Don't settle. As with all matters of the heart, you'll know when you find it" (Stanford 2005).

When you find yourself without meaning or purpose, you will know that you are in a dire situation of spiritual depletion. In the exercise below, you will have the opportunity to learn more about your level of spiritual nourishment.

EXERCISE: **Is Your Spirit Well Nourished?**

1. From the list of spiritual depletion signs below, checkmark the ones that you currently experience.

   ☐ melancholy or despair

   ☐ feeling tired for no reason

   ☐ hopelessness

   ☐ a lack of joy

   ☐ inability to make decisions

   ☐ chronic negativity

☐ addiction or abuse of alcohol or drugs

☐ feeling alone and isolated

☐ inability to accept or experience love or support from others

☐ trouble with motivation

☐ loss of purpose or passion

☐ restlessness

☐ feeling apathetic—as if nothing matters anymore

☐ nothing makes you happy anymore

☐ other: _____

2. What is the cause of your spiritual depletion?

☐ chronic stress

☐ grief or loss

☐ chronic illness in yourself or a loved one

☐ sudden change in life

☐ trauma—either past or present

☐ other: _____

☐ other: _____

☐ other: _____

3. If you feel you are trying to fill a hole or void, ask yourself, *To what degree and for how long did these attempts to fill the hole work, or did they work at all?* Describe how you feel about using people, behaviors, or substances to try to fill the hole. (*Example: I remember being so excited when I was on my last diet, and feeling that way for a few weeks as everyone complimented me on how much weight I'd lost. Then after all the attention went away, I still felt the same as I had before I'd lost the weight.*)

_____

_____

_____

4. If you feel you are in a pattern of always being restless, needing to make changes, ask yourself, *What about this has worked for me, and what has not?* Describe any insights you have about how this pattern leads to soul depletion and how that has affected your life. (*Example: I was unhappy in my marriage and blamed my husband for the problems. I divorced him and now am a single parent, which is much more difficult than I expected. I am in a new relationship and having some of the same issues come up that came up in my marriage.*)

    _____

    _____

    _____

5. If you identify with hopelessness as a sign of spiritual depletion, list below the things in your life that usually make you feel hopeful. Describe the event or situation that has led to hopelessness. If you feel ready, ask yourself if you can let go of what is causing you to feel hopeless and make a commitment to access things that help you feel hopeful on a daily basis. If you are not yet ready, see the next question. (*Example: When my partner of ten years died unexpectedly, I felt like I lost my way. Usually being with my kids, going to church, and being in nature fill me with hope. Right now, my hopelessness stems from the feeling of being all alone. I think I have isolated myself, and if I can just bring myself to get back in touch with the many friends we shared and spend time with my kids, I will start to heal.*)

    _____

    _____

    _____

6. If you feel you are not ready to let go of your current hopelessness or the situation that has caused it, see if you can think of three steps you can take to help you resolve this situation. Here are some ideas:

    ☐ Seek professional counseling.

☐ Seek out a minister or priest who can provide counseling.

☐ Journal about what you are feeling.

☐ Make a pros-and-cons list for letting go versus not letting go.

☐ Other: _____

☐ Other: _____

☐ Other: _____

7. If you feel you've lost your passion for life or your purpose, describe below the incident(s) that caused you to lose your passion or purpose, what you felt about this situation, and what thoughts you had that changed your passion or purpose. Next, ask yourself what it would take for you to get your passion or purpose back. How could you restore yourself to wholeness? (*Example: After I was fired from my job, I felt angry, and I was also afraid that I would no longer be able to support my family. I thought that no one would want someone who'd been fired or someone who is my age and that I was damaged goods. What it would take for me to get my purpose and passion back is to start believing in myself again.*)

_____

_____

_____

_____

_____

8. What have you learned from these past experiences that you can use now? (*Example: I've finally realized and admitted to myself that I can't fix the inside problem with something from the outside. I can't solve my loneliness and trust issues by just switching partners.*)

_____

_____

_____

_____

_____

Hopefully you can see how important it is to be aware not only of your physical and emotional health but also your spiritual health and the patterns that contribute to spiritual depletion. In the next part of this chapter, you will learn about what you can do to replenish your spirit.

Nourishing Your Spirit

Nourishing your spirit is not something you learned to do in school. You probably weren't even taught it at home. Nourishing your spirit is not an intellectual form of learning only—or at least it shouldn't be. It should be a daily practice. For example, you can read a book about meditation, but that won't give you the changes in your brain that meditating will. But if you do something every day, even if only for a short time each day, you will build a strong foundation to face life's many challenges, rather than using sandbags in the middle of a flood of stress to shore up your depleted resources. If you have a daily ritual, it can improve your overall psychological well-being and reduce anxiety. For example, meditating only twelve minutes a day for eight weeks can improve your mood, decrease fatigue, and lower your level of anxiety (Anastasi and Newberg 2008; Moss et al. 2012).

Some of the most commonly used methods to nourish your spirit include complementary and alternative medicine (CAM) therapies. If you've gotten a massage, taken vitamins or supplements, practiced breathing exercises, gone to a yoga class, seen a chiropractor, or meditated in the past twelve months, you are part of the over 40 percent of people who have used CAM therapies for stress reduction, illness, pain, anxiety, and depression (Barnes, Bloom, and Nahin 2008). Having some sort of spiritual practice (including prayer) is the most common CAM therapy used in our society, and newer research shows that if you have a spiritual practice, it can have a beneficial effect on your health. In fact, most medical schools now teach that there is a strong connection between spirituality and health. Nourishing your spirit involves the use of daily spiritual practices. Practices that inspire awe and involve acts of forgiveness tap into your passion and offer times for contemplation and relaxation (Harrington 2014). CAM therapies can offer many of these benefits, as can walks in nature and speaking with a close friend. The following sections describe other practices you can use to nourish your spirit.

The Practice of Forgiving

Forgiveness is central to many religions and spiritual traditions. The practice of forgiveness can lead to higher self-esteem, lower depression and anxiety (Hebl and Enright 1993), and better life satisfaction (Hargrave and Sells 1997). Your health may be improved through the practice of forgiveness for a variety of reasons: forgiveness enhances spirituality, reduces stress, helps with conflict management, and most importantly, helps with emotional regulation—especially of negative emotions such as anger and depression (Lawler et al. 2005).

Previously, you learned about how judgments can keep you stuck in unproductive relationships with others and with yourself. If you are too enmeshed in judgments, you will not be able to forgive yourself or others for perceived or actual harms. Forgiveness doesn't mean that you think abuses, traumas, or hurts are right or good or that they should have happened. When you forgive someone, you are giving up thoughts of retribution and also letting go of any negative charge or emotions associated with the past event. When you forgive yourself, you are giving up self-blame associated with past misdeeds or regrets about the past events (Toussaint et al. 2001). Forgiveness is something you do for yourself to free yourself from suffering. You may also realize that the person hardest to forgive is yourself. The "Forgiveness and Self-Love Meditation," a guided audio meditation available at http://www.newharbinger.com/32127, will help you begin to let go of experiences that block your ability to be forgiving and loving.

In the upcoming exercises, you will be given a choice of different daily practices. Remember, don't try to do everything all at once or take on too much. Life is a process, not a destination. Schedule in your calendar what you want to focus on each day. You can alternate different practices, or you can choose one to focus on for a week or a month and then switch to something different. Choose things that are doable given your lifestyle and based on what you feel drawn to doing.

EXERCISE: **I Forgive You.**

List below the ways in which not forgiving others or yourself has affected your life. (*Example: My lack of forgiveness has cut me off from my daughter and my granddaughter.*)

_____

_____

_____

_____

Next, specifically list ways you would be willing to forgive yourself for any harms you've done to yourself related to your battle with food and weight issues. Some examples are listed to get you started.

- I forgive myself for the crazy diets I've put my body on.

- I forgive myself for the excessive exercise that I've engaged in.

- I forgive myself for starving myself to lose weight.

- I forgive myself for the negative self-talk I've had in the past about my body.

- I forgive myself for: _____

- I forgive myself for: _____

- I forgive myself for: _____

Daily Practice

1. Keep a journal that lists people (including yourself) who you feel have harmed you. Ask yourself what you need to do to be ready to forgive that person or yourself. On a daily basis, rate your level of readiness to forgive. Keep checking in with yourself to see what benefit you will reap by forgiving that person or yourself and how it will harm you to continue to withhold forgiveness. At the end of each week, list whom you have forgiven. For anyone you are struggling to forgive, including yourself, ask yourself, *What help do I need in order to lessen this burden?* It may be seeing a therapist or talking to your priest.

2. Choose a ritual that helps you forgive.

   ☐ Light a candle each day and say a prayer that you will be able to forgive.

   ☐ Put the names of people you want to forgive on scraps of paper and burn the names after you feel you have forgiven them.

☐ Plant a seed for a flower, herb, or other plant in a "forgiveness garden" that you can water and reflect on each day or each week.

☐ Other: _____

☐ Other: _____

3. Write an affirmation that describes your intent for practicing forgiveness. (*Example: I forgive others and myself to release the bonds that keep me from the freedom I deserve.*)

_____

_____

The Practice of Gratitude

In studies, the practice of gratitude is consistently linked with overall well-being. If you focus on things you are grateful for on a daily basis, you will be more likely to feel better about your life and will feel more optimistic. You may also exercise more and have fewer medical problems (Harvard Mental Health Letter 2011). Gratitude can also contribute to feeling happier and having better social relationships. If you are a grateful person, someone who sees gratitude as a permanent part of your personality, rather than just a temporary state of mind, you will also be more likely to take better care of yourself and engage in healthy behaviors such as exercise, eating a healthy diet, and getting regular medical checkups. Being able to feel gratitude even in the midst of trying or stressful times helps you cope better with stress (Emmons and McCullough 2003). For example, after September 11, 2001, studies showed a marked increase in feelings of gratitude even in the face of tremendous tragedy. Gratitude helped offer a buffer for people against the negative effects of trauma, making those who experienced gratitude less likely to suffer from post-traumatic stress disorder (Peterson and Seligman 2004).

Gratitude felt internally can certainly improve your overall well-being. But as William Arthur Ward said, "Feeling gratitude and not expressing it is like wrapping a present and not giving it" (BrainyQuote 2015). There is a whole spectrum of ways in which you can express your gratitude—everything from a simple thank-you and writing a note of gratitude to meeting with people from your past and letting them know how much they have contributed to your life.

In the exercise below, identify experiences you can use to cultivate gratitude.

EXERCISE: **Opportunities for Gratitude**

Below is a list of situations you may have experienced, and perhaps at the time you did not think about being grateful. If this specific situation didn't happen to you, think of others that are similar and list those.

- things my parent has done for me recently

- the last time someone opened a door for me

- things my spouse or significant other has done for me or for our family

- an act of kindness from a stranger or acquaintance

- times when I've received emotional support from a friend or acquaintance

- things coworkers have done to help me

- unexpected contributions of money, time, or support

- things in nature I'm grateful for

- pets I'm grateful for

- other: _____

- other: _____

- other: _____

- other: _____

- other: _____

- other: _____

In the exercise below, explore things you can do daily to *practice* gratitude.

EXERCISE: **Thank You**

List below areas of your life where you feel you are struggling to be grateful. *(Example: My mother does lots of thoughtful things for me, but I rarely show my appreciation.)*

_____

_____

_____

_____

In response to the list above, write specific actions you are willing to take to show your gratitude to people in the areas you listed.

_____

_____

_____

_____

Daily Practice

Choose from the list below or make your own list of things you can do every day to practice gratitude.

- Take a few minutes at the start or end of each day to take three deep breaths—breathing in gratitude with each breath and feeling the energy of gratitude pulsing throughout your body with each beat of your heart.

- Say grace before your meals.

- Say thank you to at least five people every day for one week.

- Write a thank-you note once a day for something special someone has done for you.

- Write three things every evening before bedtime that you feel grateful to yourself for (self-gratitude). Do this for one month.

- Make a collage or drawing of all the things in your life you already have and are grateful for.

- Find one thing each day that you are grateful to your body for doing for you.

- Other: _____

- Other: _____

The Practice of Living Mindfully

Living consciously, or mindfully, involves developing a focused awareness of the present moment. It is the best way to replenish your spirit. You don't need to be spiritual or religious to live mindfully. If you want to slow your pace and reduce distractions and chaos in your life, then this is the antidote to the overstimulation. Studies now show that mindful practices, such as meditation and present-moment awareness, can change the expression of genes that cause inflammation in the body and can improve your recovery from stressful events (Algeria-Torres, Baccarelli, and Bollati 2011). If you are more mindful in your daily life, you may have a better ability to regulate your emotions and you may feel more emotionally stable throughout the day. You will also sleep better because mindfulness reduces the flight-or-flight activation of the nervous system, allowing you to be more relaxed at bedtime. There is also evidence that if you live mindfully, even if you have attachment problems as discussed previously, you will be more satisfied in your romantic relationships and less likely to break up. This effect is due to the benefits of mindfulness for emotional regulation (Bei et al. 2013; Davidson et al. 2003; Prakash et al. 2013). Living mindfully can also help you with impulsivity, a trait associated with emotional and compulsive overeating and drug and alcohol abuse (Staiger et al. 2014).

Mindfulness can have a direct impact on reducing emotional eating and bingeing (Levin et al. 2014), and it may also help you lose weight (Katterman et al. 2014; O'Reilly et al. 2014). In the exercise below, work on identifying and trying one of the many ways to live more mindfully.

EXERCISE: **Living a Conscious, Mindful Life**

Take three deep breaths, eliminate distractions, and sit in a comfortable chair. Then complete the sentence fragments below by listing three responses for each one.

1. If I were to live more mindfully, I would:

    a. _____

    b. _____

    c. _____

2. When I think about my food and body image issues, if I were to live more mindfully, I would:

    a. _____

    b. _____

    c. _____

Daily Practice

Choose one of the following practices to enhance your ability to live mindfully. Before you begin, remember to use your breathing to ground yourself and focus your mind. Put your focus on your breath, noticing your breath going into your body and then noticing your breath as you exhale. Just allow any thoughts or distractions to pass by without any attention being put on them, like leaves on a stream—you watch your thoughts go by, but you don't have to do anything about them.

- Choose one of the actions you wrote down above as a daily practice.

- Practice walking meditation. Walk slowly through nature, making a point to pay attention to your surroundings like a toddler would. When your mind wanders, bring it back to the beauty in nature.

- Take a little mind trip. Daydream about someplace you've been or want to go and imagine what you will do there—what you will wear, eat, and so forth.

- Practice taking three deep breaths before starting each meal.

- Sit quietly and listen to soothing music.

- Practice listening to someone you care about and paying attention to his or her words, expressions, and emotions, without letting your mind wander.

- Get a massage and stay present with how you feel.

- Set up a home altar where you place sacred items. Light a candle each evening and sit quietly next to your altar to quiet your thoughts.

- Get up early enough to watch the sunrise.

- Other: _____

In this chapter, you've explored ways to nourish your spirit. Keeping spiritually fit is just as important as keeping physically fit and can offer the same types of benefits to your health and well-being. This is no different than what you should do to care for yourself physically and emotionally. For example, the SIMPLE plan gives you five simple recommendations to use on a daily basis to guide you in making food choices. It may seem that there is so much to do to make the necessary changes to your lifestyle, and this may seem overwhelming. However, it can help to just think of something else you've accomplished that has been complicated or required your commitment. For example, if you are a parent, you know that every day you have to feed the baby or help your toddler eat, you have to clothe her, get her buckled safely in her seat belt, provide her with discipline and support, and many other things. If you're not a parent, think of a work project that you may have completed that had many facets, timelines, multiple people involved, and other components. Sometimes we just do what needs to be done because we are already committed. The same is true with adding practices to nourish your spirit. This chapter has provided you with many good reasons why you should commit to small daily practices for spiritual nourishment. Rather than look at the long list, remind yourself to choose one small thing that you can do that makes you feel uplifted, not burdened, and that you can imagine yourself doing. This is the way great changes start—not like the diets you've been on in the past where you've had to clean all your kitchen cabinets and eat only lettuce for a month. Rather, great, long-lasting changes start when you take small steps, moving in a direction that you are attracted to, doing something you would love to do, and committing to living mindfully in just one small way.

Staying connected to your spiritual essence can help you accomplish all of your other goals for healing. Each time you take time to connect to your spirit, you will find yourself enlivened and empowered to face the challenges of your daily life.

CHAPTER 10

Finding Your Anchor

Anita started gaining weight after the birth of her first child. She was over one hundred pounds above her ideal weight. She felt her husband was no longer attracted to her, and even if he was, she didn't want to undress in front of him. Besides being overwhelmed as the mother of three young children, she was very stressed by her work. She was working as a paralegal, and although she found her work challenging and she liked the people she worked with, she didn't want to go to work in the mornings, and she couldn't wait until weekends came. As she worked through the Anchor Program and started losing weight, she realized that she had blamed most of her unhappiness on her weight. When she reflected on her level of soul satisfaction, she realized that she had left behind her dream of becoming a psychologist. As she came to understand more of the reasons she gained weight, she felt very inspired to work with other people who had the same issues. She realized that her dream job was not being a paralegal and that her lack of soul satisfaction at work was affecting other areas of her life and contributing to her weight problem. The quote on my website really resonated with her: "Being anchored is about being true to yourself and accessing your inner strength." She felt that in her work, she was not being true to herself, and she began to make plans to go back to school to become a psychologist.

In this chapter, you will work on finding your anchor. For Anita, it was her career, but it could be any area of your life where you are not experiencing soul satisfaction. It could be your family or your children or the work you do for your church. Your anchor is what keeps you going through all the tough times. It's a form of self-expression that is an integral part of who you are. In this chapter, you will have the chance to take a journey into your imagination. You will write a script about someone who is the star of his or her own show or movie—you.

Like the heroes and heroines in famous stories and movies, each of us is the hero of our own life's story. Seen from this vantage point, the question should not be, how can I lose weight? but rather, what is my spirit being called to do or change? In this chapter, you will learn why your weight and body image concerns have distracted you from your authentic self's potential for full self-expression. You will also learn how to find your own path to healing. Self-expression and soul satisfaction are the preliminary steps and the strongest anchors to help you end your struggles with weight and body dissatisfaction.

Your Hero's Journey

Joseph Campbell was an American author and teacher who studied the power of myths from around the world, finding that myths from different cultures were all the same story— just retold in different ways. He discovered that all of these stories followed the same pattern, with the hero myth being the foundation. Stories based on the hero or heroine myth have appeal to all of us because we can identify with someone struggling to overcome great odds and better him- or herself. Campbell described what is called the arc of the hero's journey—a model that has been used in many famous movies to describe the stages, conditions, and results of any mythical hero's journey through life.

If you think about it, your life has its own heroic qualities. Just as heroes in the movies have done, you too have overcome challenges in your life and you have experienced both pain and suffering and have lived to tell about it. You may even be at a point in your life where you are teaching other people to overcome similar challenges. However, you, like many heroes, may feel less than heroic because of what you consider your own personal flaw—your weight and body image issues. If not for your weight, you may think, *I could be or do anything I wanted.* You may think that if you could just lick your weight problem, you could have a better life. Again, all heroes have challenges, some of which are pivotal in their life—things they have to overcome in order to really live the life they were meant to live and find their true anchor. The crux of any life worth living is being able to be fully expressive. So, it's not the weight that has to change—it's your focus on the weight. It's not about your body size or shape—it's how you perceive your body size and shape and how you allow your body size to limit your self-expression.

The exercises in this chapter are based on Joseph Campbell's arc of the hero's journey (Campbell 1949), starring you as the hero or heroine. You will be able to identify the stages of your own journey, hopefully becoming more aware with each stage of the powerful direction your life has taken and of the magnificence of the spirit in you (your authentic self) that has conquered so much and brought you this far. Below are the stages of the hero's journey that Campbell wrote about and a short description of each stage.

1. The *ordinary world* is whatever your current life looks like. Your ordinary world shows crucial details about you as the main character—such as where you work, what your outlook on life is, what kind of person you are, and what has made you who you are today. This part of the story can also include background history, such as incidents from childhood. Overall, the ordinary world helps us see the hero (you) as a human, just like us.

2. The *call to adventure* is the beginning of the journey. This can be a threatening situation such as a health challenge, being fired at work, a breakup of a relationship, or anything that made you, for example, purchase this book. It could be something dramatic or something simple like a phone call or a conversation. Whatever happened, it disrupts your ordinary world and puts you on the journey.

3. During the *refusal of the call*, you may refuse to make a change in your life because of stubbornness or you may be afraid of moving out of your comfort zone. Refusing the call leads to more suffering, however, and will eventually make you miserable enough to start on your path.

4. The *meeting the mentor* stage occurs when you become so upset about this call to action, this disruptive situation in your life, that you seek help, whether it be purchasing a book, seeing a therapist, or getting support from a friend or family member. The mentor(s) you seek out may have gone through something similar to what you are experiencing and can help you do something you may have always been afraid to do.

5. *Crossing the threshold* is the time when you actually commit to your journey—whether you go willingly or are pushed. It may involve doing something you have been afraid to do or have been putting off, or leaving the comfort of your home or family for the first time. It is the start of your commitment.

6. You may have noticed that sometimes things get worse before they get better. These are *tests, allies, and enemies.* Along your journey, you will have to sort out whom you can trust. Sometimes, the tests you face prepare you for something bigger that will happen later. This is the stage where your skills will be tested and your trials have the potential to make you a stronger person.

7. When you *approach the innermost cave*, you reach "the wall," where you come up against an inner conflict that makes you want to quit and go back to your comfort zone. This can be a time when you reflect on what lies ahead of you on the journey and find the courage to go on.

8. The *ordeal* can be a deep inner crisis that you have to face in order to survive, or it may involve standing up to a person who has ruled or ruined your life. You have to face this ordeal in order to be reborn into the new life you so desire. In this stage, everything you hold dear will be put to the test. If you get through this stage, your life will never be the same.

9. The *reward* comes after you defeat the enemy (usually your own worst fears) and overcome your greatest personal challenge. It can come in the form of knowledge, insight, or even reconciliation with a loved one. The reward will help you return to the ordinary world and will prepare you for the last part of your journey, which is still ahead.

10. The *road back* is the return home with your reward in tow. At this stage, you may have to choose between your own personal goals and a higher cause or calling.

11. The *resurrection* stage may involve facing your last and most dangerous challenge. This last challenge represents something far greater than your small self's goals, and the outcome will have far-reaching consequences in the ordinary world and the lives of those you left behind. This may put a lot of responsibility on your shoulders, but once you conquer this challenge, you will have vanquished whatever your enemy is and emerged a different person, with soul satisfaction.

12. Finally, you *return with the gift.* After your journey to healing, you will come back home a changed person; you will have grown as a person and learned many things, and will be able to look forward to the start of a new life. The gift you bring back will represent change, success, and proof that you have conquered all the blocks on your journey.

If you're having any trouble identifying how this applies to you, think of your favorite movie and see if you can identify the different stages above in the main character's story in the movie. Epic movies such as *Star Wars* follow this pattern. Luke Skywalker starts out as the bored farm boy and then is asked to join the quest to save the world. Now, think of your own life. Maybe you grew up with abusive parents or you grew up lonely as an only child, and then something happened, such as the death of a loved one or loss of a job, that made your life change. Or you may have been diagnosed with a chronic illness or just moved to a new city to start a job. Then the journey began. In the exercise below, see if you can write the story of your personal hero's journey. Put as much detail in as possible, and use the stages above to guide you in writing your story. Try to identify ways in which your journey has led you to where you are today with your weight and body image issues and may lead you even further along the path to healing your weight and body image issues. Try to step back, as if your life story is a movie and you are watching it on the big screen. Leave out self-defeating judgments and negative thoughts about your body. Try to see your body as perfect for the leading character (you) in the movie. How have your weight and body image issues helped propel you on your own path to healing?

EXERCISE: **Your Hero's Journey**

In the sections below, describe to the best of your ability where you are at this moment in time on your journey to healing. You can project whatever parts of your journey are incomplete, creating that path in your imagination. You can be as creative as you want, writing it as a fairy tale or writing it as a true grit novel. The sections below are there to guide you, but you can also just write out a story on a different sheet of paper. You can write it based on a timeline sequence or use an event sequence. Be creative and enjoy the process!

1. My ordinary world looked like: *(Example: I was the youngest of five children, and both my parents were obese. I was put on my first diet when I was only five. I was*

teased in school because of my weight. By eighth grade, I was in a vicious cycle of dieting and overeating that led to my weighing over two hundred pounds by the time I graduated high school.)

_____

_____

_____

_____

_____

2. The calls to adventure I remember were: *(Example: The first call was after my grandmother died when I was eighteen. She was someone who really encouraged me and loved me no matter what. I tried to lose weight after her death because I realized that life really is short and I should be who I really want to be. But I was not success-ful. When I turned thirty, I was diagnosed with a serious medical problem. Two years later, I was a divorced mother of two, and I finally realized that I had to take better care of myself or my children would be alone.)*

_____

_____

_____

_____

_____

3. I refused the calls at first because: *(Example: I put everyone else first. I was also afraid that if I put myself first, I would lose the people I loved, like my spouse. I also knew that dieting was the easy way out and that I needed to work on other issues in my life, and I was afraid to do that.)*

_____

_____

_____

_____

_____

_____

4. Mentors who have helped me along the way include: *(Example: My grandmother was a mentor for me. I had a teacher in grade school who was very kind to me.)*

_____

_____

_____

_____

_____

5. The event or situation that finally pushed me to begin my journey to healing was: *(Example: When I was passed over for a promotion at work, my hopes for moving up the corporate ladder fell by the wayside, and I began to question what was really important in my life.)*

_____

_____

_____

_____

_____

6. Some of the tests, trials, friends, and foes I've met along the way include: *(After I was divorced, I was financially bankrupt, without any help from my spouse. I had just started to go back to school to get my MBA but had to quit because I couldn't support my kids and go to school. I was devastated.)*

_____

_____

_____

_____

_____

_____

7. I hit the wall in my journey when: *(Example: I hit the wall when I spoke with one of my MBA classmates who had finished his degree and I realized that ten years had gone by without my going back to school.)*

_____

_____

_____

_____

_____

_____

8. The biggest ordeal I've had to face was: *(Example: My biggest ordeal was having to stand up to my mother's criticism when I decided to go back to finish my degree, which meant I could no longer help her financially. She was angry and didn't speak to me for almost a year. I thought we were close but realized that she is very self-centered and only approves of me when I'm doing what she wants me to do.)*

_____

_____

_____

_____

_____

_____

9. The lessons I've learned and the rewards I've obtained from my journey include: (*Example: I learned that I'm much stronger than I ever thought I was. I realized that by putting myself first, I am more able to take care of my family and those I love. I know that I am a worthwhile and lovable person who doesn't have to be a people-pleaser to have love in my life.*)

_____

_____

_____

_____

_____

_____

10. Challenges I've faced later in my journey (just when I thought I was out of the woods) include: (*Example: My daughter needed a medical procedure, and I almost quit school because I didn't think I could afford both. Instead, I was able to work with her dad to get him to cover part of the cost.*)

_____

_____

_____

_____

_____

_____

11. How my experiences have changed me and changed my life: *(Example: I am no longer afraid to say no to things that I don't want or need to do. I am clear about who my real friends are and whom I can trust.)*

_____

_____

_____

_____

_____

_____

12. The gifts that I have brought back with me (knowledge, insight, stronger character) include: *(Example: I am now working with other women, teaching them how to become financially stable. In hindsight I can see my experiences have made me stronger and given me insight that I can share with other women.)*

_____

_____

_____

_____

_____

Finding Your Anchor

Hopefully, you have been able to see yourself as the hero of your own journey. No matter what stage you feel you are currently on, you have the ability to continue to create what comes next. One of the things that will help you stay on your path is finding your anchor. Being anchored is about being true to yourself and accessing your inner strength. Being anchored is the thing that keeps you going through the steps on your hero's journey. Use the next exercise to help you identify your anchor.

EXERCISE: **Finding Your Anchor**

Identify the anchor(s) in your life that keep you grounded and able to put one foot in front of the other.

1. When times get tough, the anchor(s) that keeps me going include

    a. my children or family

    b. my spiritual or religious beliefs

    c. my commitment to my career

    d. my desire to keep improving my life

    e. my spouse

    f. other: _____

    g. other: _____

    h. other: _____

Your anchor should be tied to your authentic self's soul satisfaction. While you can use your anchor to just get you through suffering, the best use is to help take you out of suffering. In previous chapters, you've learned that the authentic self is all about doing what is in your highest and best interest. The small self is focused on more superficial goals that bring you attention, recognition, and acknowledgment and wants to fix or improve your life for these purposes. In the exercise below, put your anchor(s) to good use by identifying areas of your life that would benefit from the use of your authentic self's wise knowledge.

EXERCISE: **Anchoring Yourself in Soul Satisfaction**

Take three deep breaths, and, putting your attention on the inner sensations of your feet, imagine what would be different in your life if you lived from soul satisfaction. See if you can imagine at least three ways in which your life would change. (*Example: If I were to live for soul satisfaction, I would be more gentle and less critical with myself.*)

- If I were to use my anchor(s) for soul satisfaction, I would: _____

_____

- If I were to use my anchor(s) for soul satisfaction, I would: _____

_____

- If I were to use my anchor(s) for soul satisfaction, I would: _____

_____

In the space below, make a commitment to yourself that incorporates how you will use your anchors for soul satisfaction that you can use as a "mission statement" going forward. (*Example: I commit to being kinder with myself and using my inner strength to nurture and heal my past wounds.*)

_____

_____

_____

_____

You are the hero of your own life. Each person and situation that you experience on your hero's journey is part of what has made you who you are today. There is power in embracing the movie that is your life rather than allowing it to pass by unacknowledged. When you look back on your life and see yourself as the hero or heroine, you can feel the power of that role pulsing through your entire body, washing away fear and enabling you to truly own your past. The trials and tribulations on your journey can strengthen your resolve and mold your character. There are gifts in even the most painful experiences as long as you stay anchored, being true to yourself and accessing your inner strength.

CHAPTER 11

The Seven-Week Guide to Soul Satisfaction

I n the last chapter, you found yourself being the hero or heroine of your own journey to healing from food and body image issues. The purpose of seeing yourself in this role is to take some of the shame, guilt, blame, and pain away from food and weight issues you may have been struggling with. If you can see yourself in a new light, as someone going through a process, and if you can see that all the challenges and what you may have called failures along the way are just part of that journey, it may help you recognize that what's ahead on your journey is up to you and is all part of your process. This may give you the motivation to keep going, knowing there is a gift you will return with (besides just a healthy body). The gift could be one of more self-love or compassion, or it could spark a change in your career or improve your relationships. The gift is all part of changing your focus from the number on the scale to the development of soul satisfaction.

This chapter presents a seven-week guide to help you focus your energy and attention on the different aspects of the Anchor Program that will bring you the most benefit and take you even farther down your path to true healing from your food, weight, and body image issues. Please continue to journal about your progress, about any insights you have, and about any emotions that you experience in response to this process. If you write even just a little bit each day, you can look back and see the progress you've made. Each week, you will have a suggested approach to physical activity, nutrition, and nourishing your spirit and body image. There will also be a lifestyle focus each week and an affirmation for the week. I recommend that you put your weekly affirmation in your smartphone or computer calendar with an alarm that reminds you of the affirmation each morning. Let's get started!

Week 1: Next Steps

Weekly Theme: Focus on being aware of when you are hungry and when you are full.

Dietary Goal for the Week: Keep a diet diary every day. Check how well you're doing with the SIMPLE plan.

Affirmation for the Week: Unconditional love is the greatest gift I can give others and myself.

Skill to Practice This Week: Push away negative and self-defeating thoughts by imagining them in a lockbox or writing them down on slips of paper and then burning the paper at the end of the week.

Nourish Your Spirit: Drink a cup of green tea in the morning, sitting where you can see or be in nature.

Lifestyle Focus: What support do you need this week? Find an accountability partner who will remind you to be your best self.

Physical Activity: Move your body for fun and relaxation without counting the time. Try walking, swimming, dancing, or whatever makes you feel happy!

Complementary and Alternative Medicine: Try the amino acid taurine. Taurine increases bile production, thereby improving fat metabolism (Xu et al. 2008). Taurine also reduces anxiety (Kong et al. 2006). Dosage: 1000 mg per day. *Taurine is considered safe for most people at this dosage, for up to one year. Very high doses (14 grams) should not be used if you've been diagnosed with bipolar disorder.*

The goal of week 1 is for you to continue the excellent progress you've been making with all the exercises in the previous chapters by using this guide to focus your efforts. This week should reinforce the changes you've already made and help motivate you to follow the suggestions from earlier chapters that you have not implemented. Each of the recommendations is meant to provide you with a structure that you can focus on. Keeping a journal of what you eat, how well you're following the SIMPLE plan, and how much activity you're getting is important to your overall progress toward the goal of reaching and maintaining a healthy weight and learning to eat and move with joy. This week, remember to also record how hungry you are before and after each meal. You can use a one-to-ten scale, with one being so hungry you "feel like passing out" and ten being "too stuffed to move." This is how you develop your own personal guidelines rather than relying on those experts we talked about in previous chapters. Then, move on to week 2, where you will be learning about detoxing.

Week 2: Detox

Weekly Theme: Detox your diet. Choose one eating habit you'd like to change and work on that this week. For example, you could cut out sugar (for a whole week!). Or you could try to avoid processed food.

Dietary Goal for the Week: Drink extra water this week and add fresh lime or lemon to your water. Focus on eating lots of brightly colored organic fruits and vegetables (especially broccoli), beans, and whole grains.

Affirmation for the Week: I effortlessly drop habits that no longer serve me.

Skill to Practice This Week: Learn to relax: take a detoxifying Epsom salt bath (bubbles optional) or get a massage this week.

Nourish Your Spirit: Focus on your breath. For five minutes each day, breathe in to the count of four and exhale to the count of seven. Imagine each breath bringing in peace and calm and each exhalation letting out tension, pain, and stress.

Lifestyle Focus: Spend some time in nature every day, even if only for five minutes.

Physical Activity: Work up a sweat for at least fifteen minutes each day doing anything you love!

Complementary and Alternative Medicine: Drink a detox tea every morning (see below). Help your body detox by sweating it out in a sauna or steam room.

The focus of week 2 is detoxing the body. Every day we are exposed to toxins in our environment. If you are not eating organic foods, you may also be exposed to toxic pesticides in your food. Ancient medical traditions have long extolled the virtues of periods of detoxing either by juice fasting or simply by eating foods that help your body rid itself of toxins. Drinking extra water will help flush toxins out of the body, as will working up a sweat and going to a sauna or steam room. Adding lemon or lime to your water improves your digestive processes and helps with elimination. The most important foods you can eat when you are detoxing are fruits and vegetables. Make a "detox shake" for breakfast that contains carrots, beets, kale, ginger, and pea protein. Double your portion of raw and lightly cooked vegetables. Add a handful of kale, collards, or spinach to soup. Eating foods high in anti-oxidants, such as organic fruits and vegetables, helps activate liver enzymes that get rid of harmful substances (Curl, Fenske, and Elgethun 2003; Hennig et al. 2012). Examples of super antioxidants include spinach, kale, and cranberries. Broccoli and other cruciferous vegetables contain nutrients that help neutralize and eliminate toxins in the body natu-rally (Peterson et al. 2005). Detox teas are sold in most health food stores and are generally recognized as safe to use and usually contain dandelion, which supports digestion and liver function (WebMD 2014); licorice, which expels mucus and reduces body fat (Armanini et al. 2003; University of Maryland 2015); and ginger, which has been traditionally used to stimulate circulation and help with stomach upset (Howe 2014). However, if you are preg-nant or taking medications, you should check with your physician before using.

One reason to spend a week detoxing your body is to be able to identify the effect of certain foods on your body when you start using them again. This is not about some foods being "bad" for you and others being "good." Eliminating a food group from your diet for a week will enable you to see how certain foods affect you. For example, you may find that mixing certain foods together causes indigestion. Or you may find that cutting out pro-cessed foods reduces sugar cravings. We'll talk more about cravings later in this chapter, but for now, if you are craving sweets, try eating fruits and vegetables in their place. Remember, you can use this week to detox from caffeine, gluten, sugar, or processed foods.

If you feel motivated, you can extend your detox to two or three weeks. When you finish your detox experience, reintroduce foods in their natural state and see if you can sustain eating fewer processed foods. Notice how you feel at the end of the week, and journal about any insights you may have. For example, you may notice that you mainly want to eat sweets when you feel anxious or bored, or you may find that you have fewer cravings when you eat more fruits and vegetables.

Most importantly, make sure you get enough fiber with each meal while detoxing. You can take an over-the-counter fiber supplement or just focus on eating more fruits and veg-etables, all of which are high in fiber. If you find you are constipated, drink extra water and take a fiber supplement before each meal. You can also take a magnesium supplement (450–900 mg at bedtime) safely, which will help reduce constipation.

Week 3 will focus on stress management and how to eat, move, and live in ways that help you manage your stress more effectively.

Week 3: Stress Management

Weekly Theme: Destress your diet and your life.

Dietary Goal for the Week: Eat foods high in B vitamins, such as asparagus, avocados, and green leafy vegetables (spinach, kale, collard greens). Add garlic to your diet. Snack on cashews and walnuts. Eliminate caffeine and alcohol for one week.

Affirmation for the Week: Today I create a stress-free world for myself when I let my thoughts come from the loving space of my own heart, where forgiveness and nonjudgment emanate.

Skill to Practice this Week: Self-soothing for stress reduction: put on lavender lotion, listen to relaxing music, or savor a piece of dark chocolate.

Nourish Your Spirit: Share a meal. Cook a meal at home and invite people you care about to dine with you, or put together a potluck.

Lifestyle Focus: Quiet the mind. Sit quietly for sixty seconds, allowing your thoughts to pass by and your mind to become quiet. Increase the time by one minute each day.

Physical Activity: Try a mindful exercise such as yoga, Pilates, tai chi, or qigong. You can rent a DVD from your local library or take a class at the gym.

Complementary and Alternative Medicine: Get an acupuncture treatment. Drink ginseng tea in the morning. Take a B-complex vitamin.

You've learned about stress in previous chapters, and the focus here should be on practicing what you've learned and applying it to your diet and lifestyle. Good nutrition can help you fight the negative effects of stress on the body. Supplements such as B-complex vitamins and omega-3 fatty acids or foods high in these nutrients will also help you fight stress. B vitamins (B-complex) are important in nerve cell health and support of mood. B vitamins are necessary in the production of feel-good brain chemicals (neurotransmitters) such as serotonin, dopamine, norepinephrine, and epinephrine. If you are a strict vegetarian or vegan, you may have vitamin B-12 deficiency. Deficiencies can also result from some medications (including medications for acid reflux). Foods high in B vitamins include fortified breakfast cereals, fish, pork, chicken, bananas, beans, peanut butter, and many vegetables, including dark green leafy vegetables. You can also get a B-complex vitamin from your health food store. Another food to consider is one you may think has no place in a "healthy diet." (This is yet another reason to never be on a diet again!) I'm referring to dark chocolate, which is high in antioxidants and also helps support good mood. Just eat a small square and enjoy every single bite.

Other ways to manage stress include physical activity and learning ways to soothe yourself without food. Think of using your five senses to self-soothe, and try different experiences to see what works best for you. Social support is another way to cope with stress. Eating a delicious meal with friends or doing another activity that puts you out in your community, such as volunteering, are also ways to help manage stress. If you haven't tried acupuncture, you may consider visiting your local traditional Chinese medicine school to get a (usually reduced-fee) treatment or consult a seasoned acupuncturist, which can help reduce the activation of your nervous system caused by stress.

Another tip is to drink ginseng tea. Ginseng is an "adaptogen" (Shergis et al. 2013), which helps your body deal with stress, as discussed in chapter 8.

Week 4: Addressing Cravings

Weekly Theme: Dealing with cravings for foods and the desire to want things in your life to be as they are not.

Dietary Goal for the Week: Eat protein at every meal and snack. Protein helps balance the diet and reduce food cravings.

Affirmation for the Week: Gratitude unlocks the fullness of life. Today I am grateful for all that I have and all that I am.

Skill to Practice This Week: Practice riding the waves of your emotions. Cravings will pass if you wait them out and don't act on them. Wait ten minutes before you give in to cravings. Ask yourself: *Is this craving coming from my body or from my mind and emotions? What do I really need right now?* Try to provide yourself with your true need rather than giving in to cravings.

Nourish Your Spirit: Get a good night's (seven to nine hours) sleep. Sleeping well makes you less vulnerable to emotional eating.

Lifestyle Focus: Journal about your feelings. See if you can identify patterns associated with your cravings. Write at least one paragraph a day this week to just get your feelings out of your head and onto the page.

Physical Activity: Moving your body is a great way to "let off steam" emotionally and to help you manage your mood. Physical activity also helps your brain make better decisions, be less impulsive, and say no to your cravings.

Complementary and Alternative Medicine: Eat bitter foods to reduce sweet cravings (see below). For salt cravings, address causes of stress and use adaptogens such as ginseng (Shergis et al. 2013). The mineral chromium stabilizes blood sugar (Ryan et al. 2003) and reduces cravings (Docherty et al. 2005).

Many people struggle with cravings for sweet, salty, or fatty foods. By being aware of what you are feeling (rather than numbing or ignoring your feelings), you are more likely to be able to interrupt the cycle of emotional overeating. Journaling about what you are feeling is a good way to identify whether you are hungry physically versus emotionally. Physical hunger usually has signs such as a growling stomach, headache, or even light-headedness. Emotional hunger is usually associated with obsessive or racing thoughts about a particular food, agitation, anxiety, depression, or other mood changes. When you find yourself considering eating a box of cookies or a large bag of chips, you know this isn't physical hunger. When you are aware of this, you can ask yourself the questions above. You may not know right away what your need is, but if you keep asking the questions, you will be able to tap into your body's wisdom to help you determine whether you need a hug or someone to talk to or just some alone time. Even if you give in to the cravings, try to eat mindfully and pay attention to how your body is feeling. If your journaling shows that you're always hungry (emotionally) after stressful days at work, change your routine. Don't go straight home and binge on peanut butter; stop at a local park and take a short walk, or call a friend to meet you for tea.

Traditional Chinese medicine suggests the use of bitters to combat sugar cravings. Bitters can be purchased as a tincture from the health food store or you can eat foods that have a bitter quality—such as endive, radicchio, cooked greens, and olives. The mineral chromium helps reduce cravings by stabilizing blood sugar. Infection, pregnancy, stress, or a diet high in sugar can cause chromium deficiency. Talk to your health care provider about taking a chromium supplement if you crave sweets. Salt cravings may indicate adrenal fatigue caused by stress. Chronic dieting and overconsumption of sweets and starchy foods or processed foods puts extra stress on your adrenal glands, so your body is less able to respond to stress effectively. So if you're craving salty foods, work on reducing your stress through yoga, meditation, breathwork, and the use of ginseng tea.

Finally, getting a good night's sleep has multiple benefits, including improved mood and reduced emotional eating. People who sleep less than seven to nine hours a night are more likely to be overweight or obese (Gangwisch et al. 2005). Good sleep habits include sleeping in a darkened room that is quiet and using your bedroom only for sleep or sex. Don't leave the television on while you are trying to fall asleep. Good sleep helps with stress reduction and is important for overall good health.

Week 5: Enhancing Your Energy Level

Weekly Theme: Reclaim your energy. Foods that increase energy are discussed below.

Dietary Goal for the Week: Monitor portion sizes using the fist-and-palm method and plating your food on a nine-inch plate. Overeating can sap your energy.

Affirmation for the Week: I love myself exactly as I am. I no longer wait to be perfect in order to love who I am.

Skill to Practice This Week: Practice mindfully eating three meals and one snack at the same times each day. Set alarms on your phone to remind you to stop what you are doing and take time to eat mindfully.

Nourish Your Spirit: Listen to inspiring spiritual teachers' recordings—for example, Eckhart Tolle, Pema Chodron, and Deepak Chopra. Play them on your commute to work.

Lifestyle Focus: Where are you blocking your energy flow by holding on to past hurts, toxic emotions, and limiting beliefs? What can you do to open up your energy channels to abundance, joy, and positivity? Journal about these questions this week.

Physical Activity: Get a pedometer to count the number of steps you take during the day. The more steps you take, the more energy you will have. Shoot for ten thousand steps a day.

Complementary and Alternative Medicine: If you have trouble falling asleep, add a few drops of vanilla essential oil to a tissue and put the tissue inside your pillowcase.

Not having enough energy or feeling tired is a common problem. You may be one of the 20 percent of people who have even gone to see a doctor with a complaint of fatigue (Rosenthal et al. 2008). Fatigue can be caused by medical problems such as low thyroid and low iron (in women who are premenopausal), but most commonly, it is related to lifestyle factors such as what you eat, how much you sleep, how active you are, and how much stress or emotional upheaval you have in your life. You've learned about stress and sleep in this and previous chapters. What you may not know is that what you eat can either enhance or decrease your energy levels. In general, foods that tend to promote good, sustainable energy include protein-rich foods. These foods are also good sources of iron and include poultry and meats along with lentils and beans, spinach, and eggs. Too little iron can lower your metabolic rate and your energy. If you are a premenopausal woman, you may know that you lose iron each month with your menstrual cycle, and if your diet does not contain enough iron (18 mg per day), you may become anemic (low in iron), leading to fatigue. Dehydration is another cause of low energy, so be sure you drink enough water. The main thing is not to limit certain foods or even to eat more or certain foods. The most important thing you can do is to just notice how different types of foods affect your energy level. For example, if you find yourself exhausted by midmorning, look back at what you ate for breakfast (or did you skip breakfast?). Then experiment to find out the perfect combination for *you* to improve your overall energy.

If you feel tired during the day, take advice from an old, yet oft-quoted study and take just a ten-minute brisk walk, which is more energizing than eating a candy bar. Walking also increases energy for a longer (two hours) period of time (Thayer 1987). Drinking caffeine when you're exhausted may make you feel wired without boosting energy and can interrupt your sleep cycle, so use caffeine with caution. To keep your energy up, stick with eating good sources of protein, fruits, and vegetables; drinking lots of water; and moving your body.

Week 6: Good Gut Function

Weekly Theme: Pay attention to your gut and notice how it feels with the different foods you eat.

Dietary Goal for the Week: Add foods that are high in probiotics, which promote gut health (see below).

Affirmation for the Week: I relax my mind and body, and I radiate joy. I am part of the harmonious whole and know all is well in my world.

Skill to Practice This Week: Practice paying attention to your "gut" or your intuitive wisdom—at work, at home, with your food, and throughout your day. See if you can identify what you are feeling about different situations, and don't let what you are thinking make you second-guess your feelings. Make notes in your journal.

Nourish Your Spirit: Practice belly breathing. Place your hands on your belly. Breathe in, expanding your belly, allowing it to collapse with the exhalation. Inhale and exhale to the count of seven. Repeat five times.

Lifestyle Focus: Increase fiber in your diet to improve gut function. See more below.

Physical Activity: Physical activity that is aerobic is helpful for gut function, as is yoga.

Complementary and Alternative Medicine: Consider an abdominal massage treatment that may help with weight loss and improve gut function.

If you have a weight issue or binge-eating disorder, you may also suffer from digestive complaints (Delgado-Aros et al. 2004), which may impair your digestion. There is a direct connection between your gut and your brain and emotions. There is a direct link between the type of bacteria in your gut and your levels of anxiety and depression (Rao et al. 2009). There is also evidence to show that obesity is linked to changes in gut flora. For this reason, I recommend you take probiotics in pill form to help you reduce digestive complaints such as gas, constipation, and bloating and to promote overall gut health (Ross, Herman, and Rojas 2008). I also recommend you include foods that contain probiotics and prebiotics in your diet. Probiotic-containing foods actually contain live bacteria, while prebiotic foods feed the bacteria already living in your gut. Probiotic-containing foods include fermented foods such as kimchi; unpasteurized sauerkraut; miso; dairy foods including yogurt, soft cheeses (gouda), and kefir; and fermented soybeans (tempeh). Prebiotics are found in foods such as asparagus, Jerusalem artichokes, bananas, red wine, honey, maple syrup, oatmeal, beans, lentils, and peas (legumes).

Probiotics supply your digestive system with bacteria that fight inflammation and improve digestion. Stress, your diet, and frequent use of antibiotics can diminish the levels of healthy bacteria in your gut. Probiotics use may also affect body weight (Blaut and Bischoff 2010; Mekkes et al. 2014).

Fiber is good for the gut. There are two types of fiber: soluble and insoluble. If you eat foods high in soluble fiber, you will feel more full, a benefit for weight loss. It also helps you lower your LDL (bad) cholesterol, keep blood sugar stable, and lower your risk for heart disease and diabetes (Seal and Brownlee 2015). If you eat foods high in insoluble fiber, you will have better elimination and relief of constipation. Foods containing soluble fiber include oatmeal, lentils, beans and peas, apples, pears, berries, nuts, carrots, cucumbers, and celery. Foods containing insoluble fiber include whole grains, dark leafy greens, raisins, zucchini, cabbage, onions, tomatoes, green beans, and broccoli. If you're like the average American, you may get only fifteen of the recommended twenty-five (women) to thirty-eight (men) grams of fiber per day. For the purposes of this week, try to increase your intake of fruits, vegetables, and legumes (beans, lentils, and peas), and try to eat only whole grains. This will give you a good mix of both soluble and insoluble fiber.

Week 7: Connecting Your Brain and Heart for Maximum Soul Satisfaction

Weekly Theme: Connection, creation, soul satisfaction

Dietary Goal for the Week: What can you add to your diet that will support you in creating the life you want?

Affirmation for the Week: I know that miracles are all around me, and I have the power to create miracles in my own life.

Skill to Practice this Week: Visioning. Take a large piece of construction paper or poster board. Next, decide on the theme for your vision board—for example, *My Healthy Life*. Or you could choose a more specific theme having to do with an aspect of what you're working on in this book, such as *Body Esteem* or *Satisfying My Soul*. Then clip out pictures from magazines, draw or paint words, or find old photographs that go along with your theme. Include some affirmations that you find inspiring. Glue everything on your board and then hang it in a place where you will see it every day. Each day, take a moment in front of the board to just look at what you've created and feel inspired by the future you're moving toward.

Nourish Your Spirit: Create a positive start to each day: Write the affirmation of the week (or another that you favor) on a piece of paper and put it next to your bed. Each morning, read the affirmation before getting up.

Lifestyle Focus: What can you do to create the life you want? Journal about areas of your life where you want to bring something into being. Is it at work, at home, or with family or friends? Write next to each one a small step you can take to begin your creation—for example, "I will sign up to take a yoga class."

Physical Activity: Identify a form of body movement that you can make a one-month commitment to doing, and make a commitment to trying this body movement activity at least once a week.

Complementary and Alternative Medicine: Develop a place in your house where you can meditate and listen to calming music, journal, or sit quietly, focusing on your breath. Decorate the area to suit your taste with candles, feathers, smooth stones, or whatever invokes a feeling of peace and relaxation.

There is a story, often attributed to a Native American source, that speaks of a youngster who goes to his grandfather and says: "I have two wolves inside of me. One wants to kill and destroy, and the other wants to bring peace and beauty. Which one will win, Grandfather?" The old man answers, "Whichever one you feed." This is such a beautiful proverb for people who are struggling with food, weight, and body image issues. Often when you are focused on the number on the scale, you are feeding the wolf that is about appearance, judgment, past hurts or traumas, and low self-esteem. Throughout this book, you have learned about all the reasons why you've come to focus on the superficial level of appearance. You've learned all about the core beliefs, emotions, and body sensations that are part of what brought you to this time in your life. You've also learned about how your childhood may have resulted in an insecure attachment style and difficulty connecting with others. It is fitting to end on the note of where you put your attention, or which wolf you will continue to feed. If you truly want to heal, you will feed the wolf that offers soul satisfaction. How do you do that?

Humans are hardwired for connection. When babies stare into the eyes of their mothers and see their love reflected back, their heart rate and brain waves entrain to that of their mothers (Feldman et al. 2011). One way to feed the wolf of soul satisfaction is to create such connections in your life now. You can create connection and spiritual support with friends, therapists or other health care providers, and family members whom you feel safe with.

In terms of your brain, the destructive wolf lives in your primitive brain, which is always in survival mode, always telling you to be afraid and to react to life situations from the fight-flight-freeze stress reaction. When your thinking can move into the higher aspects of the brain (neocortex and prefrontal cortex) and out of the primitive brain (amygdala and limbic system), you move out of fear and into joy, creativity, innovation, and a feeling of connectedness to others, to nature, and to life itself. How do you spend more time in the higher parts of your brain? Meditation, mindfulness, and breathwork all help. Mindfulness is doing anything where you are able to focus your attention only on what you are doing, closing out all distractions. This could be eating, swimming, talking to your child, dancing, having sex—anything! Meditation also benefits heart rhythms (Lee et al. 2015). Mindfulness-based stress reduction, developed by Jon Kabat-Zinn, can improve emotional regulation, learning, and memory (Center for Mindfulness 2015). Breathwork is also important for this brain shift. Notice your breathing patterns the next time you're feeling stressed, anxious, or angry, and you will find that your breathing may become more rapid and shallow. This shallow breathing, by itself, induces anxiety and panic. Concentrating on taking slow, deep breaths can lower blood pressure and induce relaxation all by itself (Mori et al. 2005).

What your brain is going through affects your heart. Feelings and thoughts of anger, frustration, and sadness actually change your heart rhythm to a more chaotic one (Taggart, Critchley, and Lambiase 2011). Feelings of appreciation and gratitude, on the other hand, create heart rhythms that are calm and peaceful (McCraty 2001). Petting your dog, sitting in nature, and talking to a friend are examples of things you can do to create these healthy heart rhythms.

Imagery is the language of your subconscious and uses your senses to invoke a future desire or goal. The last week of your seven-week program for soul satisfaction is about creating the life you want to have. You may not have had control over how you grew up or what family you were born into. Perhaps you tried to get some control back or decided unconsciously to let go of control completely through an unhealthy relationship with food. Throughout this book, you've learned why you did that, and hopefully, you've learned many reasons why you don't want to continue acting from the same patterns as before. The "Guided Imagery for Soul Satisfaction," a guided audio meditation available at http://www .newharbinger.com/32127, will help you connect brain and heart and in the process, affirm the parts of your current life you love and create a new way of being based on living from soul satisfaction.

Conclusion

You've come a long way since first opening this book! As you heal from food, weight, and body image issues, you may notice changes in your body. These changes on the outside reflect changes you are making on the inside. Remember to listen to your body's wisdom to guide your eating. Also remember that "feeling fat" is not a state of being; it is a state of mind. See if you can find room in your heart to allow your body to be just the way it is and have that be okay with you. By staying in the present moment and practicing gratitude and appreciation toward your body, you will be aligning your inside with your outside to live from a congruent, authentic place.

Everything you've done is part of what it takes to heal from food, weight, and body image issues. You should give yourself a pat on the back for working through this workbook and being willing to look at some tough issues from your past and in the present. Try not to fall back into unhealthy patterns (although you will from time to time), and when you do, just remind yourself that even this is part of the natural process of healing. Be kind to yourself. Interrupt any judgmental thoughts, and continue to foster hope and express gratitude for the arc of your personal hero or heroine's journey. You are a survivor, and now your job is to learn to thrive! You've taken some big steps in what is always the journey of a lifetime. Whatever your next steps are, I wish you health and happiness!

References

Adam, T. C., and E. S. Epel. 2007. "Stress, Eating and the Reward System." *Physiology Behavior* 91 (4): 449–58.

Agras, W. S., L. D. Hammer, F. McNicholas, and H. C. Kraemer. 2004. "Risk Factors for Childhood Overweight: A Prospective Study from Birth to 9.5 Years." *Journal of Pediatrics* 145: 20–25.

Ainsworth, M. D., M. Blehar, E. Waters, and S. Wall. 1978. *Patterns of Attachment: A Psychological Study of the Strange Situation.* Hillsdale, NJ: Lawrence Erlbaum Associates.

Algeria-Torres, J. A., A. Baccarelli, and V. Bollati. 2011. "Epigenetics and Lifestyle." *Epigenomics* 3 (3): 267–77.

Anastasi, M. W., and A. B. Newberg. 2008. "A Preliminary Study of the Acute Effects of Religious Ritual on Anxiety." *Journal of Alternative and Complementary Medicine* 14 (2): 163–65.

Anda, R. F., and V. J. Felitti. 2003. "Origins and Essence of the Study." *ACE Reporter* 1 (1): 1–3.

Armanini, D., C. B. De Palo, M. J. Mattarello, P. Spinella, M. Zaccaria, A. Ermolao, et al. 2003. "Effect of Licorice on the Reduction of Body Fat Mass in Healthy Subjects." *Journal of Endocrinological Investigation* 26 (7): 646–50.

Bacon, L. 2008. *Health at Every Size.* Dallas: BenBella Books.

Bacon, L., and L. Aphramor. 2011. "Weight Science: Evaluating the Evidence for a Paradigm Shift." *Nutrition Journal* 10: 9.

Baldaro, B., N. Rossi, R. Caterina, M. Codispoti, A. Balsamo, and G. Trombini. 2003. "Deficit in the Discrimination of Nonverbal Emotions in Children with Obesity and Their Mothers." *International Journal of Obesity* 27: 191–95.

Barnes, P. M., B. Bloom, and R. L. Nahin. 2008. "Complementary and Alternative Medicine Use Among Adults and Children: United States, 2007." *National Health Statistics* 12: 1–23.

Bechara, A., H. Damasio, and A. Damasio. 2000. "Emotion, Decision Making and the Orbitofrontal Cortex." *Cerebral Cortex* 10 (3): 295–307.

Bei, B., M. L. Byrne, C. Ivens, J. Waloszek, M. J. Woods, P. Dudgen, G. Murray, C. L. Nicholas, J. Trinder, and N. B. Allen. 2013. "Pilot Study of a Mindfulness-Based, Multi-Component, In-School Group Sleep Intervention in Adolescent Girls." *Early Intervention Psychiatry* 7 (2): 213–20.

Belsky, J., and M. J. Rovine. 1988. "Nonmaternal Care in the First Year of Life and the Security of Infant-Parent Attachment." *Child Development* 59 (1): 157–67.

Benoit, D. 2014. "Infant-Parent Attachment: Definition, Types, Antecedents, Measurement, and Outcome." *Pediatrics and Child Health* 9 (8): 541–45.

Bentley, T., and C. S. Widom. 2009. "A 30-Year Follow-Up of the Effects of Child Abuse and Neglect on Obesity in Adulthood." *Obesity* 17 (10): 1900–1905.

Birch, L. L., and J. A. Fisher. 1995. "Attitude and Eating Behavior in Children." *Pediatric Clinics of North America* 42 (4): 931–53.

Blaut, M., and S. C. Bischoff. 2010. "Probiotics and Obesity." *Annals of Nutrition and Metabolism* 57 Suppl: 20–23.

Boisvert, J. A., and W. A. Harrell. 2013. "The Impact of Spirituality on Eating Disorder Symptomatology in Ethnically Diverse Canadian Women." *International Journal of Social Psychiatry* 59 (8): 729–38.

Boudarene, M., J. J. Legros, and M. Timsit-Berthier. 2002. "Study of the Stress Response: Role of Anxiety, Cortisol and DHEAs." *Encephale* 28 (2): 139–46.

BrainyQuote. 2015. "William Arthur Ward Quotes." Accessed July 29, 2015. http://www.brainyquote.com/quotes/quotes/w/williamart105516.html.

Brown, D. W., R. F. Anda, H. Tiemeier, V. J. Felitti, V. J. Edwards, J. B. Croft, and W. H. Giles. 2009. "Adverse Childhood Experiences and the Risk of Premature Mortality." *American Journal of Preventative Medicine* 37: 389–96.

Brown, G. W., T. O. Harris, and C. Hepworth. 1995. "Loss, Humiliation and Entrapment Among Women Developing Depression: A Patient and Non-Patient Comparison." *Psychological Medicine* 25: 7–21.

Burkeman, O. 2009. "The Bedsit Epiphany." *The Guardian.* Accessed August 5, 2015. http://www.theguardian.com/books/2009/apr/11/eckhart-tolle-interview-spirituality.

Campbell, J. 1949. *The Hero with a Thousand Faces.* Novato, CA: New World Library.

Cash, T. F., J. Theriault, and N. M. Annis. 2004. "Body Image in an Interpersonal Context: Adult Attachment, Fear of Intimacy and Social Anxiety." *Journal of Social and Clinical Psychology* 23 (1): 89–103.

CDC (Centers for Disease Control and Prevention). 2014. "The Benefits of Physical Activity." Accessed June 18, 2014. http://www.cdc.gov/physicalactivity/everyone/health/.

Center for Mindfulness. 2015. "Stress Reduction." Accessed August 17, 2015. http://www.umassmed.edu/cfm/stress-reduction/.

Chen, M. C., S. H. Fang, and L. Fang. 2013. "The Effects of Aromatherapy in Relieving Symptoms Related to Job Stress Among Nurses." *International Journal of Nursing Practice* 21 (1): 87–93.

Cho, J. H., S. Y. Jae, I. L. Choo, and J. Choo. 2014. "Health-Promoting Behaviour Among Women with Abdominal Obesity: A Conceptual Link to Social Support and Perceived Stress." *Journal of Advanced Nursing* 70 (6): 1381–90.

Coccia, C., and C. A. Darling. 2014. "Having the Time of Their Life: College Student Stress, Dating and Satisfaction with Life." *Stress Health.* doi: 10.1002/smi.2575

Corstorphine, E., V. Mountford, S. Tomlinson, G. Waller, and C. Meyer. 2007. "Distress Tolerance in the Eating Disorders." *Eating Behaviors* 8: 91–97.

Curl, C. L., R. A. Fenske, and K. Elgethun. 2003. "Organophosphorus Pesticide Exposure of Urban and Suburban Preschool Children with Organic and Conventional Diets." *Environmental Health Perspectives* 111 (3): 377–82.

Davidson, R. J., J. Kabat-Zinn, J. Schumacher, M. Rosenkranz, D. Muller, S. Santorelli, et al. 2003. "Alterations in Brain and Immune Function Produced by Mindfulness Meditation." *Psychosomatic Medicine* 65 (4): 564–70.

Davis, C., W. B. Dutton, T. Durant, R. A. Annunziato, and D. Marcotte. 2014. "Achieving Cultural Congruency in Weight Loss Interventions: Can a Spirituality-Based Program Attract and Retain an Inner-City Community Sample?" *Journal of Obesity*. doi: 10.1155/2014/641939

De Schipper, J. C., M. Oosterman, and C. Schuengel. 2012. "Temperament, Disordered Attachment and Parental Sensitivity in Foster Care: Differential Findings on Attachment Security for Shy Children." *Attachment and Human Development* 14 (4): 349–65.

Delgado-Aros, S., G. R. Locke III, M. Camilleri, N. J. Talley, S. Fett, A. R. Zinsmeister, and L. J. Melton III. 2004. "Obesity Is Associated with Increased Risk of Gastrointestinal Symptoms: A Population-Based Study." *The American Journal of Gastroenterology* 99: 1801–6.

Dittman, K. A., and M. R. Freedman. 2009. "Body Awareness, Eating Attitudes, and Spiritual Beliefs of Women Practicing Yoga." *Eating Disorders* 17 (4): 273–92.

Docherty, J. P., D. A. Sack, M. Roffman, M. Finch, and J. R. Komorowski. 2005. "A Double-Blind, Placebo-Controlled, Exploratory Trial of Chromium Picolinate in Atypical Depression: Effect on Carbohydrate Craving." *Journal of Psychiatric Practice* 11 (5): 302–14.

Du, S., Y. Tao, and A. M. Martinez. 2014. "PNAS Plus: Compound Facial Expressions of Emotion." *Proceedings of the National Academy of Sciences of the USA* 11 (15): E1454–62.

Ekman, P., W. V. Friesen, and P. Ellsworth. 1982. "What Emotion Categories or Dimensions Can Observers Judge from Facial Behavior?" In *Emotion in the Human Face*, edited by P. Ekman, 39–55. New York: Cambridge University Press.

Emmons, R. A., and M. E. McCullough. 2003. "Counting Blessings Versus Burdens: An Experimental Investigation of Gratitude and Subjective Well-Being in Daily Life." *Journal of Personality and Social Psychology* 84 (2): 377–89.

Everson, S. A., G. A. Kaplan, D. E. Goldberg, and J. T Salonen. 2000. "Hypertension Incidence is Predicted by High Levels of Hopelessness in Finnish Men." *Hypertension* 35: 561–67.

Feldman, R., R. Magori-Cohen, G. Galili, M. Singer, and Y. Louzoun. 2011. "Mother and Infant Coordinate Heart Rhythms Through Episodes of Interaction Synchrony." *Infant Behavior and Development* 34: 569–77.

Felitti, V. J., R. F. Anda, D. Nordenberg, D. F. Williamson, A. M Spitz, V. Edwards, M. P. Koss, and J. S. Marks. 1998. "Relationship of Childhood Abuse and Household Dysfunction to Many of the Leading Causes of Death in Adults. The Adverse Childhood Experiences (ACE) Study." *American Journal of Preventative Medicine* 14: 245–58.

Fox, N. A., and A. A. Hane. 2008. "Studying the Biology of Human Attachment." In *Handbook of Attachment: Theory, Research and Clinical Applications*, edited by J. Cassidy and P. R. Shaver, 811–29. New York: Guilford Press.

Frankl, V. 1992. *Man's Search for Meaning*. Boston: Beacon Press.

Gangwisch, J. E., D. Malaspina, B. Boden-Albala, and S. B. Heymsfield. 2005. "Inadequate Sleep as a Risk Factor for Obesity: Analyses of the NHANES I." *Sleep* 28 (10): 1289–96.

Gianini, L. M., M. A. White, and R. M. Masheb. 2013. "Eating Pathology, Emotion Regulation and Emotional Overeating in Obese Adults with Binge Eating Disorder." *Eating Behaviors* 14 (3): 309–13.

Gillath, O., P. R. Shaver, J. M. Baek, and D. S. Chun. 2008. "Genetic Correlates of Adult Attachment Style." *Personality and Social Psychology Bulletin* 34 (10): 1396–405.

Goldschmidt, A. B., J. R. Best, R. I. Stein, B. E. Saelens, L. H. Epstein, and D. E. Wilfley. 2014. "Predictors of Child Weight Loss and Maintenance Among Family-Based Treatment Completers." *Journal of Consulting Clinical Psychology*. doi: 10.1037/a0037169

Greeno, C. G., and R. R. Wing. 1994. "Stress-Induced Eating." *Psychological Bulletin* 115: 444–64.

Haatainen, K. M., J. K. Tanskanen, J. Kylma, K. Honkalampi, H. Kolvumaa-Honkanen, J. Hinitkka, and H. Viinamaki. 2004. "Factors Associated with Hopelessness: A Population Study." *International Journal of Social Psychiatry* 50: 142–52.

Haedt-Matt, A., and P. Keel. 2011. "Revisiting the Affect Model of Regulation of Binge Eating: A Meta-Analysis of Studies Using Ecological Momentary Assessment." *Psychological Bulletin* 137: 660–81.

Haeffel, G. J., B. E. Gibb, G. I. Metalsky, L. B. Alloy, L. Y. Abramson, B. L. Hankin, T. E. Joiner Jr., and J. D. Swendsen. 2008. "Measuring Cognitive Vulnerability to Depression: Development and Validation of the Cognitive Style Questionnaire." *Clinical Psychology Review* 28 (5): 824–36.

Hall, J. A., and D. Matsumoto. 2004. "Differences in Judgments of Multiple Emotions from Facial Expressions." *Emotion* 4 (2): 201–6.

Hargrave, T., and J. Sells. 1997. "The Development of a Forgiveness Scale." *Journal of Marital and Family Therapy* 23: 41–62.

Harrington, A. 2014. "Health and Spirituality." Accessed July 23. http://nccam.nih.gov /training/videolectures/spirituality.htm.

Harvard Mental Health Letter. 2011. "In Praise of Gratitude." Harvard Health Publications. Accessed August 8, 2015. http://www.health.harvard.edu/newsletter_article/in-praise -of-gratitude.

Haslam, M., V. Mountford, C. Meyer, and G. Waller. 2008. "Invalidating Childhood Environments in Anorexia and Bulimia Nervosa." *Eating Behaviors* 9 (3): 313–18.

Hebl, J., and R. Enright. 1993. "Forgiveness as a Psychotherapeutic Goal with Elderly Females." *Psychotherapy* 30: 658–67.

Hendricks, G., and K. Hendricks. 1993. *Centering and the Art of Intimacy Handbook: A New Psychology of Close Relationships.* New York: Fireside Books.

Hennig, B., L. Ormsbee, C. J. McClain, B. A. Watkins, B. Blumberg, L. G. Bachas, W. Sanderson, C. Thompson, and W. A. Suk. 2012. "Nutrition Can Modulate the Toxicity of Environmental Pollutants: Implications in Risk Assessment and Human Health." *Environmental Health Perspectives* 120 (6): 771–74.

Howe, M. 2014. "Warm Up to Ginger." WebMD. Accessed November 30, 2014. http:// www.webmd.com/food-recipes/features/warm-up-to-ginger.

Hu, Elise. 2012. "'Seventeen' Magazine Takes No-Photoshop Pledge After 8th-Grader's Campaign." NPR. Accessed June 10, 2014. http://www.npr.org/blogs/thetwo-way /2012

/07/05/156342683/seventeen-magazine-takes-no-photoshop-pledge-after-8th-graders-campaign.

Insel, T. R., and L. J. Young. 2001. "The Neurobiology of Attachment." *Nature Review Neuroscience* 2 (2): 129–36.

Integral Yoga Magazine. 2009. "Yoga and Post-Traumatic Stress Disorder." *Integral Yoga Magazine Summer,* 12–13. Accessed August 4, 2015. http://www.integralyogamagazine.org/yoga-and-post-traumatic-stress-disorder.

Kanayama, G., S. Barry, J. I. Hudson, and H. G. Pope. 2006. "Body Image and Attitudes Toward Male Roles in Anabolic-Androgenic Steroid Users." *American Journal of Psychiatry* 163: 697–703.

Katterman, S. N., B. M. Kleinman, M. M. Hood, L. M. Nackers, and J. A. Corsica. 2014. "Mindfulness Meditation as an Intervention for Binge Eating, Emotional Eating and Weight Loss: A Systematic Review." *Eating Behavior* 15 (2): 197–204.

Kennedy, D. O., J. L. Reay, and A. B. Scholey. 2007. "Effects of 8 Weeks Administration of Korean Panax Ginseng Extract on the Mood and Cognitive Performance of Healthy Individuals." *Journal of Ginseng Research* 31: 34–43.

Kong, W. X., S. W. Chen, Y. L. Li, Y. J. Zhang, R. Wang, L. Min, and X. Mi. 2006. "Effects of Taurine on Rate Behaviors in Three Anxiety Models." *Pharmacology Biochemistry and Behavior* 83 (2): 271–76.

Larsen, J. K., T. van Strien, R. Elsinga, and R. C. Engels. 2006. "Gender Differences in the Association Between Alexithymia and Emotional Eating in Obese Individuals." *Journal of Psychosomatic Research* 60 (3): 237–43.

Lawler, K. A., J. W. Younger, R. L. Piferi, R. L. Jobe, K. A. Edmondson, and W. H. Jones. 2005. "The Unique Effects of Forgiveness on Health: An Exploration of Pathways." *Journal of Behavioral Medicine* 28 (2): 157–67.

Lawson, R., F. Emmanuelli, J. Sines, and G. Waller. 2008. "Emotional Awareness and Core Beliefs Among Women with Eating Disorders." *European Eating Disorders Review* 16 (2): 155–59.

Leary, M. R., and J. P. Price. 2012. *Handbook of Self and Identity*, 2nd ed. New York: Guilford Press.

Lee, Y. H., Y. J. Shiah, S. C. Chen, S. F. Wang, M. S. Young, and C. L. Lin. 2015. "Improved Emotional Stability in Experienced Meditators with Concentrative Meditation Based on Electroencephalography and Heart Rate Variability." *Journal of Alternative and Complementary Medicine* 21 (1): 31–39.

Leung, N., G. Waller, and G. Thomas. 2000. "Outcome of Group Cognitive-Behavior Therapy for Bulimia Nervosa: The Role of Core Beliefs." *Behaviour Research and Therapy* 38 (2): 145–56.

Levin, M. E., K. Dalrymple, S. Himes, and M. Zimmerman. 2014. "Which Facets of Mindfulness Are Related to Problematic Eating Among Patients Seeking Bariatric Surgery?" *Eating Behavior* 15 (2): 298–305.

Linehan, M. M. 1993. *Cognitive-Behavioral Treatment of Borderline Personality Disorders*. New York: Guilford Press.

Lissau, I., and T. I. A. Sorensen. 1995. "Parental Neglect During Childhood and Increased Risk of Obesity in Young Adulthood." *The Lancet* 343 (8893): 324–27.

Main, M., and J. Solomon. 1986. "Discovery of an Insecure Disoriented Attachment Pattern: Procedures, Findings and Implications for the Classification of Behavior." In *Affective Development in Infancy*, edited by T. Brazelton and M. Youngman. Norwood, NJ: Ablex.

Mann, T., A. J. Tomiyama, E. Westling, A. M. Lew, B. Samuels, and J. Chatman. 2007. "Medicare's Search for Effective Obesity Treatments: Diets Are Not the Answer." *American Psychology* 63 (3): 220–33.

Marsiglia, F. F., S. Kulis, H. Garcia Perez, and M. Bermudez-Parsai. 2011. "Hopelessness, Family Stress, and Depression Among Mexican-Heritage Mothers in the Southwest." *Health and Social Work* 36 (1): 7–18.

Matsumoto, D., D. Keltner, M. N. Shiota, M. G. Frank, and M. O'Sullivan. 2008. "What's in a Face? Facial Expressions as Signals of Discrete Emotions." In *Handbook of Emotions*, edited by M. Lewis, J. M. Haviland, and L. Feldman Barrett, 211–34. New York: Guilford Press.

McCraty, R. 2001. "Psychophysiological Coherence: A Proposed Link Among Appreciation, Cognitive Performance, and Health." Accessed August 17, 2015. https://www.heart math.org/assets/uploads/2015/02/Psychophysiological-Coherence-A-Proposed-Link .pdf.

McDougall, J. 1989. *Theaters of the Body: A Psychoanalytic Approach to Psychosomatic Illness.* New York: W. W. Norton and Company.

McKinley, N. M., and L. A. Randa. 2005. "Adult Attachment and Body Satisfaction. An Exploration of General and Specific Relationship Differences." *Body Image* 3: 209–18.

Mekkes, M. C., T. C. Weenen, R. J. Brummer, and E. Claassen. 2014. "The Development of Probiotic Treatment in Obesity: A Review." *Beneficial Microbes* 5 (1): 19–28.

Merriam-Webster Online, s.v. "emotion." Accessed August 4, 2015. http://www.merriam -webster.com/dictionary/emotion.

Miller, L., R. Bansal, P. Wickramaratne, X. Hao, C. E. Tenke, M. M. Weissman, and B. S. Peterson. 2014. "Neuroanatomical Correlates of Religiosity and Spirituality: A Study in Adults at High and Low Familial Risk for Depression." *JAMA Psychiatry* 71 (2): 128–35.

Mitchell, K. S., A. M. Dick, D. M. DiMartino, B. N. Smith, K. C. Koenen, and A. Street. 2014. "A Pilot Study of a Randomized Controlled Trial of Yoga as an Intervention for PTSD Symptoms in Women." *Journal of Trauma Stress* 27 (2): 121–28.

Mori, H., H. Yamamoto, M. Kuwashima, S. Saito, K. Hirao, M. Yamauchi, and S. Umemura. 2005. "How Does Deep Breathing Affect Office Blood Pressure and Pulse Rate?" *Hypertension Research* 28 (6): 499–504.

Moss, A. S., N. Wintering, H. Roggenkamp, D. S. Khalsa, M. R. Waldman, D. Monti, and A. B. Newberg. 2012. "Effects of an 8-Week Meditation Program on Mood and Anxiety in Patients with Memory Loss." *Journal of Alternative Complementary Medicine* 18 (1): 48–53.

Mountford V., E. Corstorphine, S. Tomlinson, and G. Waller. 2007. "Development of a Measure to Assess Invalidating Childhood Environments in the Eating Disorders." *Eating Behaviors* 8 (1): 48–58.

Myers, J. 2003. "Exercise and Cardiovascular Health." *Circulation* 107: e2–e5.

Nam, S. 2013. "Effects of Social Support and Spirituality on Weight Loss for Rural African-American Women." *ABNF Journal* 24 (3): 71–76.

National Organization for Women. 2012. "NOW Foundation Releases Survey Results on 15th Birthday of Love Your Body Day." Accessed June 10, 2014. http://now.org/media

-center/press-release/now-foundation-releases-survey-results-on-15th-birthday -of-love-your-body-day/.

Niedenthal, P. M., S. Krauth-Gruber, and F. Ric. 2006. *Psychology of Emotion: Interpersonal, Experiential, and Cognitive Approaches*. New York: Psychology Press, 305–42.

O'Reilly, G. A., L. Cook, D. Spruijt-Metz, and D. S. Black. 2014. "Mindfulness-Based Interventions for Obesity-Related Eating Behaviors: A Literature Review." *Obesity Review* 15 (6): 453–61.

Pace, U., M. Cacioppo, and A. Schimmenti. 2012. "The Moderating Role of Father's Care on the Onset of Binge Eating Symptoms Among Female Late Adolescents with Insecure Attachment." *Child Psychiatry and Human Development* 43 (2): 282–92.

Pate, R. R., M. P. Pratt, S. N. Blair, W. L. Haskell, C. S. Macera, C. Bouchard, et al. 1995. "Physical Activity and Public Health: A Recommendation from the Centers for Disease Control and Prevention and the American College of Sports Medicine." *JAMA* 273: 402–7.

Paulson, S., R. Davidson, A. Jha, and J. Kabat-Zinn. 2013. "Becoming Conscious: The Science of Mindfulness." *Annals of the New York Academy of Sciences* 1303: 87–104.

Paykel, E. S., and Z. Cooper. 1992. "Life Events and Social Stress." In *Handbook of Affective Disorders*, edited by E. S. Paykel, 149–70. New York: Guilford Press.

Perry, B. D. 2009. "Examining Child Maltreatment Through a Neurodevelopmental Lens: Clinical Applications of the Neurosequential Model of Therapeutics." *Journal of Loss and Trauma* 14: 240–55.

Peselow, E., S. Pi, E. Lopez, A. Besada, and W. W. Ishak. 2014. "The Impact of Spirituality Before and After Treatment of Major Depressive Disorder." *Innovative Clinical Neuroscience* 11 (3–4): 17–23.

Peterson, C., and M. E. P. Seligman. 2004. *Character Strengths and Virtues: A Handbook and Classification*. Washington, DC: American Psychological Association.

Peterson, S., J. Bigler, N. K. Horner, J. D. Potter, and J. W. Lampe. 2005. "Cruciferae Interact with the UGT1A1*28 Polymorphism to Determine Serum Bilirubin Levels in Humans." *Journal of Nutrition* 135: 1051–55.

Pinaquy, S., H. Chabrol, C. Simon, J-P Louvet, and P. Barbe. 2003. "Emotional Eating, Alexithymia, and Binge-Eating Disorder." *Obesity* 11 (2): 195–201.

Prakash, S., A. A. De Leon, M. Klatt, W. Malarkey, and B. Patterson. 2013. "Mindfulness Disposition and Default-Mode Network Connectivity in Older Adults." *Social Cognitive Neuroscience* 8 (1): 112–17.

Rao, A. V., A. C. Bested, T. M. Beaulne, M. A. Katzman, C. Iorio, J. M. Berardi, and A. C. Logan. 2009. "A Randomized, Double-Blind, Placebo-Controlled Pilot of a Probiotic in Emotional Symptoms of Chronic Fatigue Syndrome." *Gut Pathology* 1: 6.

Reas, D. L., C. M. Grilo, R. M. Masheb, and G. T. Wilson. 2005. "Body Checking and Avoidance in Overweight Patients with Binge Eating Disorder." *International Journal of Eating Disorders* 37: 342.

Ricca, V., G. Castellini, C. Lo Sauro, C. Ravaldi, F. Lapi, E. Mannucci, C. M. Rotella, and C. Faravelli. 2009. "Correlations Between Binge Eating and Emotional Eating in a Sample of Overweight Subjects." *Appetite* 53 (3): 418–21.

Rosenthal, T. C., B. A. Majero, R. Pretorius, and K. Malik. 2008. "Fatigue: An Overview." *American Family Physician* 78 (10): 1173–79.

Ross, C. C., P. Herman, and J. Rojas. 2008. "Integrative Medicine for Eating Disorders." *Explore: The Journal of Science and Healing* 4 (5): 315–20.

Ryan, G. J., N. S. Wanko, A. R. Redman, and C. B. Cook. 2003. "Chromium as Adjunctive Treatment for Type 2 Diabetes." *Annals of Pharmacotherapy* 37 (6): 876–85.

Saarni, C. 1999. *The Development of Emotional Competence.* New York: Guilford Press.

Satter, E. M. 2008. *Secrets of Feeding a Healthy Family.* Madison, WI: Kelcy Press.

Savage, J. S., J. O. Fisher, and L. L. Birch. 2007. "Parental Influence on Eating Behavior: Conception to Adolescence." *Journal of Law, Medicine and Ethics* 35 (1): 22–34.

Schmid, G., A. Schreier, R. Meyer, and D. Wolke. 2010. "A Prospective Study on the Persistence of Infant Crying, Sleeping and Feeding Problems and Preschool Behaviour." *Acta Paediatrica* 99: 286–90.

Seal, C. J., and I. A. Brownlee. 2015. "Whole-Grain Foods and Chronic Disease: Evidence from Epidemiological and Intervention Studies." *Proceedings of the Nutrition Society* 74 (3): 313–19.

Seeyave, D. M., S. Coleman, D. Appugliese, R. F. Corwyn, R. H. Bradley, N. S. Davidson, N. Kaciroti, and J. C. Lumeng. 2009. "Ability to Delay Gratification at Age 4 Years and

Risk of Overweight at Age 11 Years." *Archives of Pediatrics and Adolescent Medicine Journal* 163: 303–8.

Shalev, A. Y., S. Freedman, T. Peri, D. Brandes, T. Sahar, and S. P. Orr. 1998. "Prospective Study of Post-Traumatic Stress Disorder and Depression Following Trauma." *American Journal of Psychiatry* 155: 630–37.

Sheffield, A., G. Waller, F. Emanuelli, J. Murray, and C. Meyer. 2009. "Do Schema Processes Mediate Links Between Parenting and Eating Pathology?" *European Eating Disorders Review* 17 (4): 290–300.

Shergis, J. L., A. L. Zhang, W. Zhou, and C. C. Xue. 2013. "Panax Ginseng in Randomized Controlled Trials: A Systematic Review." *Phytotherapy Research* 27 (7): 949–65.

Siegel, D. J. 2013. *Brainstorm.* New York: Penguin Books.

Sim, L., and J. Zeman. 2006. "The Contribution of Emotion Regulation to Body Dissatisfaction and Disordered Eating in Early Adolescents." *Journal of Youth and Adolescence* 35: 219–28.

Sines, J., G. Waller, C. Meyer, and L. Wigley. 2008. "Core Beliefs and Narcissistic Characteristics Among Eating-Disordered and Non-Clinical Women." *Psychology Psychotherapy* 81 (Pt 2): 121–29.

Sominsky, L., and S. J. Spencer. 2014. "Eating Behavior and Stress: A Pathway to Obesity." *Frontiers in Psychology* 5: 434.

Spinazzola, J., A. M. Rhodes, D. Emerson, E. Earle, and K. Monroe. 2011. "Application of Yoga in Residential Treatment of Traumatized Youth." *Journal of the American Psychiatric Nurses Association* 17 (6): 431–44.

Staiger, P. K., S. Dawe, B. Richardson, K. Hall, and N. Kambouropoulos. 2014. "Modifying the Risk Associated with an Impulsive Temperament: A Prospective Study of Drug Dependence Treatment." *Addiction Behavior* 39 (11): 1676–81.

Stanford. 2005. "'You've Got to Find What You Love,' Jobs Says." Accessed August 20, 2013. http://news.stanford.edu/news/2005/june15/jobs-061505.html.

Staples, J. K., M. F. Hamilton, and M. Uddo. 2013. "A Yoga Program for the Symptoms of Post-Traumatic Stress Disorder in Veterans." *Military Medicine* 178 (8): 854–60.

Stice, E., K. Presnell, and D. Spangler. 2002. "Risk Factors for Binge Eating Onset in Adolescent Girls: A 2-Year Prospective Investigation." *Health Psychology* 21: 131–38.

Stice, E., and K. Whitenton. 2002. "Risk Factors for Body Dissatisfaction in Adolescent Girls: A Longitudinal Investigation." *Developmental Psychology* 38: 669–78.

Taggart, P., H. Critchley, and P. D. Lambiase. 2011. "Heart-Brain Interactions in Cardiac Arrhythmia." *Heart* 97 (9): 698–708.

Temple University. 2007, November 16. "Higher Risk of Obesity for Children Neglected By Parents." *ScienceDaily.* Accessed August 5, 2015. http://www.sciencedaily.com/releases/2007/11/071113100319.htm.

Thayer, R. E. 1987. "Energy, Tiredness, and Tension Effects of a Sugar Snack Versus Moderate Exercise." *Journal of Personal and Social Psychology* 52 (1): 119–25.

Thomas, S. L., J. Hyde, A. Karunaratne, R. Kausman, and P. A. Komesaroff. 2008. "They all work…when you stick to them": A Qualitative Investigation of Dieting, Weight Loss, and Physical Exercise in Obese Individuals." *Nutrition Journal* 7: 34. doi:10.1186/1475-2891-7-34.

Tolle, E. 2015. "Eckhart Tolle Quote." Good Reads. Accessed August 10, 2015. http://www.goodreads.com/quotes/177877-accept—then-act-whatever-the-present-moment-contains-accept.

Toussaint, L. L., D. R. Williams, M. S. Musick, and S. A. Everson. 2001. "Forgiveness and Health: Age Differences in a US Probability Sample." *Journal of Adult Development* 8 (4): 249–57.

Troisi, A., G. Di Lorenzo, S. Alcini, R. C. Nanni, C. Di Pasquale, and A. Siracusano. 2006. "Body Dissatisfaction in Women with Eating Disorders: Relationship to Early Separation Anxiety and Insecure Attachment." *Psychosomatic Medicine* 68: 449–53.

Tuck, I., R. Alleyne, and W. Thinganjana. 2006. "Spirituality and Stress Management in Healthy Adults." *Journal of Holistic Nursing* 24 (4): 245–53.

Turney, D., and K. Tanner. 2005. "Understanding and Working with Neglect." *Research in Practice: Every Child Matters Research Briefings* 10: 1–8.

University of Maryland. 2015. "Licorice." Accessed August 10, 2015. http://umm.edu/health/medical-reference-guide/complementary-and-alternative-medicine-guide/herb/licorice.

Unoka, Z., T. Tolgyes, and P. Czobor. 2007. "Early Maladaptive Schemas and Body Mass Index in Subgroups of Eating Disorders: A Differential Association." *Comprehensive Psychiatry* 48 (2): 199–204.

U.S. National Library of Medicine. 2014. "Gingseng, Panax." *MedlinePlus.* Accessed June 24, 2014. http://www.nlm.nih.gov/medlineplus/druginfo/natural/1000.html.

U.S. Public Health Service, Office of the Surgeon General. 1996. *Physical Activity and Health: A Report of the Surgeon General.* Atlanta, GA: U.S. Department of Health and Human Services, Centers for Disease Control and Prevention, National Center for Chronic Disease Prevention and Health Promotion.

Van der Kolk, B. A. 1994. "The Body Keeps the Score: Memory and the Emerging Psychobiology of Post Traumatic Stress." *Harvard Review of Psychiatry* 1: 253–65.

Van der Kolk, B. A. 2005. "Developmental Trauma Disorder." *Psychiatric Annals* 35 (5): 401–8.

Van der Kolk, B. A. 2006. "Clinical Implications of Neuroscience Research in PTSD." *Annals of New York Academy of Sciences* 2006: 1–17.

Van der Kolk, B. A., and R. E. Fisler. 1994. "Childhood Abuse and Neglect and Loss of Self-Regulation." *Bulletin of the Menninger Clinic* 58: 145–68.

Van Hanswijck, D. J., G. Waller, A. Fiennes, Z. Rashid, and J. J. Lacey. 2003. "Reported Sexual Abuse and Cognitive Content in the Morbidly Obese." *Eating Behaviors* 5 (4): 315–22.

Waller, G. 2003. "Schema-Level Cognitions in Patients with Binge Eating Disorder: A Case Control Study." *International Journal of Eating Disorders* 33 (4): 458–64.

Waller, G., H. Kennerley, and V. Ohanian. 2007. "Schema-Focused Cognitive Behavioral Therapy with Eating Disorders." In *Cognitive Schemas and Core Beliefs in Psychiatric Disorders: A Scientist–Practitioner Guide,* edited by L. P. Riso, P. L. du Toit, D. J. Stein, and J. E. Young, 139–75. New York: American Psychological Association.

Waters, E., and E. M. Cummings. 2000. "A Secure Base from Which to Explore Close Relationships." *Child Development* 71: 164–72.

WebMD. 2014. "Dandelion." Accessed November 30, 2014. http://www.webmd.com/vitamins-supplements/ingredientmono-706-dandelion.aspx?activeingredientid=706&activeingredientname=dandelion.

Whipple, M. O., T. T. Lewis, K. Suggon-Tyrell, K. A. Matthews, E. Barinas-Mitchell, L. H. Powell, and S. A. Everson-Rose. 2009. "Hopelessness, Depressive Symptoms and Carotid Atherosclerosis in Women: The Study of Women's Health Across the Nation (SWAN) Heart Study." *Stroke* 40 (10): 3166–72.

World Health Organization. May 2014. "10 Facts on Obesity." Accessed August 1, 2015. http://www.who.int/features/factfiles/obesity/en/.

Xu, Y-J, A. S. Ameja, P. S. Tappia, and N. S. Dhalla. 2008. "The Potential Health Benefits of Taurine in Cardiovascular Disease." *Clinical and Experimental Cardiology* 13 (2): 57–65.

Yardley, L., L. J. Ware, E. R. Smith, S. Williams, K. J. Bradbury, E. J. Arden-Close, et al. 2014. "Randomised Controlled Feasibility Trial of a Web-Based Weight Management Intervention with Nurse Support for Obese Patients in Primary Care." *International Journal of Behavioral Nutrition and Physical Activity* 11: 67.

Young, J. E., J. S. Klosko, and M. D. Weishaar. 2003. *Schema Therapy: A Practitioner's Guide*. New York: Guilford Press.

Carolyn Coker Ross, MD, MPH, is an integrated medicine physician, author, and nationally recognized speaker. She is a graduate of the University of Michigan Medical School, and an alumna of Andrew Weil's integrative medicine program at the University of Arizona. Board certified in addiction medicine, Ross is former chief of the eating disorders program at Sierra Tucson, an internationally acclaimed addiction treatment center in Tucson, AZ. She is currently in private practice in Denver, CO, and San Diego, CA, and is a consultant for the Integrative Life Center in Nashville, TN, and other eating disorder and chemical dependency treatment centers nationally. She is author of *The Binge Eating and Compulsive Overeating Workbook*.

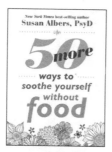
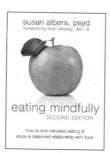
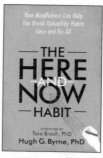
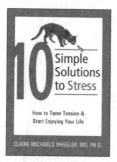
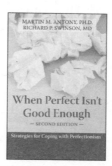
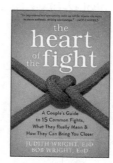
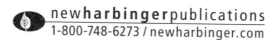

Register your **new harbinger** titles for additional benefits!

When you register your **new harbinger** title—purchased in any format, from any source—you get access to benefits like the following:

- Downloadable accessories like printable worksheets and extra content
- Instructional videos and audio files
- Information about updates, corrections, and new editions

Not every title has accessories, but we're adding new material all the time.

Access free accessories in 3 easy steps:

1. Sign in at NewHarbinger.com (or **register** to create an account).

2. Click on **register a book**. Search for your title and click the **register** button when it appears.

3. Click on the **book cover or title** to go to its details page. Click on **accessories** to view and access files.

That's all there is to it!

If you need help, visit:

NewHarbinger.com/accessories

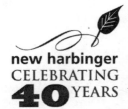

new harbinger
CELEBRATING
40 YEARS